Rise
Ever Upward

Justine Froelker

Ever Upward

Overcoming the Lifelong Losses of Infertility
to Define Your Own Happy Ending

Justine Brooks Froelker

NEW YORK

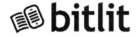 Upward

Overcoming the Lifelong Losses of Infertility to Define Your Own Happy Ending

Published in New York, New York, by Morgan James Publishing. Morgan James and The Entrepreneurial Publisher are trademarks of Morgan James, LLC.
www.MorganJamesPublishing.com

The Morgan James Speakers Group can bring authors to your live event. For more information or to book an event visit The Morgan James Speakers Group at www.TheMorganJamesSpeakersGroup.com.

bitlit

A **free** eBook edition is available
with the purchase of this print book.

CLEARLY PRINT YOUR NAME ABOVE IN UPPER CASE

Instructions to claim your free eBook edition:
1. Download the BitLit app for Android or iOS
2. Write your name in **UPPER CASE** on the line
3. Use the BitLit app to submit a photo
4. Download your eBook to any device

ISBN 978-1-63047-348-8 paperback
ISBN 978-1-63047-349-5 eBook
ISBN 978-1-63047-350-1 hardcover
Library of Congress Control Number:
2014944259

Front design image:
Kristen Ashley

Back cover photo:
Brian Brooks and Kristen Ashley

Interior Design by:
Bonnie Bushman
bonnie@caboodlegraphics.com

In an effort to support local communities, raise awareness and funds, Morgan James Publishing donates a percentage of all book sales for the life of each book to Habitat for Humanity Peninsula and Greater Williamsburg.

Get involved today, visit
www.MorganJamesBuilds.com

Habitat
for Humanity®
Peninsula and
Greater Williamsburg
Building Partner

Dedication

To Chad,

*my husband, my partner and the true witness of my ever
upward, who has always believed in my ever upward with his
empowering silent stoicism and his logical business savvy.
But mostly just by the way he loves me.*

*And to all those who suffer in shamed silence of any kind,
especially the silence of infertility, may you find and fight
for redefining your light to embrace your ever upward.*

Table of Contents

Acknowledgements

Finding my ever upward and completing *Ever Upward* was a blessing filled with ups and downs, hard work and lots of love. I could not have ever found my ever upward, let alone complete *Ever Upward* without the help, support, pushing, feedback and love from many.

First to the amazing speakers from Emerging Women, those mentioned in the coming pages and those not, you gave me the spark of magic I needed to forge forward with this project. To my friends from Emerging Women; Erica, Marie, Melinda, Michele, Sarah, Tanya, Tova, I will forever be grateful for your lights in my life.

Second to the team at The Daring Way™ and the brave women I met there, a wholehearted thank you. Thank you Brené Brown: for your work, your research and your passion. Thank you, to you and Ashley especially, for taking the time to send me a signed copy of *Daring Greatly* after the conference. It means the world. And to my fellow vulnerability warriors; Jen, Melissa, Nicole and Sabrina, thank you for the push to own myself again. And, of course for being the ones who laugh with me so hard we are asked to quiet down in a restaurant.

To my therapist Shellie, thank you for allowing me to doubt, struggle and find myself again. To my friend and colleague Kelly Tipton, thank you for your immense support through this entire journey and for asking me the hard questions I needed to find my own answers to. And to Colleen Dunford, my friend and my editor, thank you for joining me on the journey of writing *Ever Upward*. I have learned so much from you and feel so blessed that you believed in me and this enough to become part of it.

Thank you to our friends, who are truly our family, for your support throughout the IVF journey and for your love and laughter during and thereafter. Thank you for allowing us to be part of your families and always including us. There are simply not sufficient enough words other than thank you for how much it means that you not only don't forget about your childfree couple friends but find room in your families for us. Thank you especially to the Porter Family, the Schaeperkoetter Family and the Smith Family. Thank you so much to Sam and to Janine for just being some of my favorite mothers in the whole world and for allowing me to be part of that world. To Kelly, thank you for being my lifelong friend through it all and for letting me in to your own journey of finding your family. I will be forever grateful for being a part of Abigail Justine's birth and being there to watch you become a family, I love you all so much!

Thank you to my friends who have been by my side, from afar or close, on this journey back to myself. Your help, your support, your listening ears and especially your laughter have gotten me through some of the toughest times of my life. Thank you, especially for holding the space I needed to find me again. Thank you especially to Lindsay, for simply just always being my person. To Casey, thank you for always giving the insight I need and for allowing me to be such a part of McKinley's life.

Thank you to our chosen family the Ziesmer's. Thank you for your trust in embarking on the surrogacy journey with us. I am so grateful for our epic story and can't wait to see what has yet to be written in it. Michelle, thank you for your love, your spirit, and for being a true soul sister.

Thank you to my in laws, Jim and Terry. Thank you for your example of faith and your patience with me as I found and embraced mine. Thank you for all the help you've provided us throughout the years. And, thank you for your bravery in joining us in this journey. Ultimately, thank you for how you love us both.

To my parents, Brian and Linda, thank you. There is simply too much to thank you for; the moves, the manual labor, the financial help, the love, the laughter, the care. Thank you mostly for always allowing me to struggle, recover and be me. Thank you for being one of my true witnesses in life. I love you both very much.

Why Ever Upward?

"We must let go of the life we have planned,
so as to accept the one that is waiting for us."
—Joseph Campbell

The silver lining?

Excelsior?

Make the best of it?

Find your new path.

Redefine.

Ever Upward.

My story.

My story of figuring out how to stop proving that I'm okay. To stop proving that saying no more to IVF is okay. To stop proving that saying adoption isn't for us is okay. To stop proving that childless, childfree, is okay.

To stop proving it, and to really own it.

To fight for it. To figure it all out.

To truly own it. Own every part of it.

To own my ever upward.

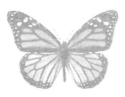

Chapter 1

Conceiving Our Chosen Family

I've spent most of my teenage and adult life convincing myself that I didn't want to be a mother. Rather than admit the hurt and loss of not being able to physically carry my own child, I emphatically said out loud that I didn't want kids. As you may have guessed, that was never met with warm and fuzzy opinions from anyone.

"You have to have kids!"

"But, you're so good with kids!"

"Oh, you'll change your mind!"

As a therapist, I know now it was all a ruse, a defense mechanism my subconscious had developed to protect me from the heartache of accepting that having children, the traditional way, just wasn't a possibility for me. Due to medical complications from high school, I knew that carrying a pregnancy was simply not something many doctors would recommend, or a risk I was willing to take. Chad and I got married, him being fully aware that children were probably not in the future for us. However, as he would later admit, he always knew we would figure out a way.

For the most part, people were right: I did change my mind. I can't tell you when or how, but just that something grew inside of me. The desire to have our own children, to see which characteristics they would get from Chad or I, my red hair and freckles or his height, my love for dance or his decathlete athletic ability, my vivacious laugh or his kind smile? The desire to set out on the hardest journey on earth with the best partner in the world. To build our family. But I knew that I could never go through a pregnancy, the risks were just too great.

While my (and Chad's) dreams of a child were growing, surrogacy was beginning to get more and more press. Celebrities were publicly sharing their story of using a surrogate to achieve pregnancy, and my world opened up. Frankly, the entire world opened up, especially through some of the surrogate message boards and blogs. Placing a simple ad on a surrogate message board, for some advice and direction on gestational surrogacy was our first step in building our family, our destined family. Little did we know our destined family didn't even include our baby.

I was overwhelmed by the immediate outpouring of love and bravery. The responses from women came in very quickly. So many women reached out just to offer words of wisdom and advice. I was completely unaware of the vast community available to those going through infertility treatments. I received several emails every day those first couple of weeks. Emails came in from women just offering support. Some offered advice, and some offered their uteruses. I was amazed at how quickly I knew that certain women just were not a good fit for us.

With some women I knew right way, such as the women who had just finished a journey with another couple (sometimes their second or third journey) and were ready to start again. I knew I wanted more from my surrogate than a quick and easy business deal. I wanted her to be more than just my internet oven. It was also easy to know when we were just too different. I trusted my instincts when our answers to the difficult questions didn't match up or our personalities were just too different to get through a year without further trauma.

The messages back and forth with women fell within the trusting space of true authentic vulnerability. You had to lay everything on the line. What do you believe in? What do you want? No reasons necessary and no apologies. Why are you doing this? Do you believe in selective reduction? What is your opinion and willingness on transferring multiple embryos? How much compensation do you want for bed rest? What kind of relationship with the surrogate family do you want after the baby is born? What about termination for special needs? All difficult questions and not ones you tend to open with upon meeting someone for the first time. I was grateful for the anonymous bravery that comes in the online world.

In February 2011, Michelle answered our ad, our prayers, our spirit and our love. She came out of nowhere, and yet from the very beginning I knew we were meant to be in each other's lives. Michelle and I built our friendship quickly through all of those difficult questions. We talked online for a couple of months before exchanging phone numbers and texting and talking. We finally got the courage to meet in person that August. Chad and I drove to Indianapolis to meet our potential surrogate and her husband. I will never forget how nervous I was. What if they weren't cool? Or funny? Or even nice? Or, what if I totally misread her intentions in doing this and feel like I can't really trust her? What if she changes her mind right then and there after meeting us and doesn't want to do this? What if they think we would be terrible parents?

We met Michelle and Ben at their favorite restaurant in their quaint town, quite possibly the cutest town in America, *Gilmore Girls* cute. It was awkward, *really* awkward, but for maybe 15 seconds. We ate, we drank wine, we laughed and we just put everything on the table. It fit, we fit; we were supposed to meet these people. In many ways it was like meeting my soul's match, there sitting across the table was my soul sister. The weekend ended in hilarity and a story that will go down in our history of our lifelong friendship and chosen family. A high school reunion, too much wine, amazing laughs and the first realization that Michelle and I are more alike than different, our hearts being more similar than just our physical red hair; it was the first of many memories of our new chosen family.

The next step before moving forward with the drugs and procedures was to meet Ben and Michelle's children. We discovered the tiny town of Effingham, Illinois, directly in the middle between Saint Louis and Indianapolis with a clean and cheap hotel with a pool for the kids to swim. It was a cold, dreary day in the fall. I remember because the kids walked Maddie and Bosco (our dogs at that time) and you can see Nathan and Lyla's (and Maddie's) hair blowing in the wind in one of my favorite pictures from our journey.

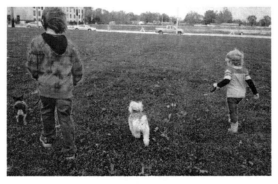

Meeting Nathan and Lyla

We ate some of the best pizza we've ever eaten before, swam, laughed and further solidified our chosen family in the little town of Effingham, IL, most infamous for the giant white cross off the highway. Michelle let us know that Nathan had an idea of who we were, but Nathan had never said anything in front of us. As for Lyla, we just became part of her extended family; little did we know she had already formed a soul mate like connection of her own with our Yorkie-poo, Maddie.

The toughest part of my friendship with Michelle was during the contract process. At the end of the day, gestational surrogacy is a business deal, not a friendship or family matter. Going back and forth with the lawyers, and not really talking much, took a toll on our friendship. The contract negotiations were difficult considering we were in different states, which therefore meant different surrogacy laws. It was confusing in the least, but also very anxiety provoking. You are paying someone to carry your baby and give birth. It is business, with a lot of money involved, but we also loved and respected these people. Chad looked at me one night and said, "I think we have to prepare that they aren't ready for this. You have to call her." I called Michelle, with my heart pounding out of my chest and a huge lump in my throat, to ask what could have been the question to end it all, "Are you sure you are ready for this and want to do this?" We had gone back and forth so many times, and gone over our attorney retainers more than once. It was one of the first times that I simply put everything on the table, even though it would have been much easier to avoid or minimize. I was scared to death that her answer might be no, that she'd changed her mind. We both cried and realized we were feeling the exact same way: torn, confused, uncomfortable and just wanting to skip over this mandatory part of the process. This is a business deal, as our husbands kept reminding us, but it was so much more. We were friends, we had started to become family, and we were both just scared shitless. It was during the contract negotiations that I felt the fear of losing them forever for the first time. What if this doesn't work out? I was scared to death of having to start over with a new surrogate. To go through the difficult questions again and find someone who believed in and would honor our wishes, felt so daunting. But this was not my greatest fear in the slightest. I was scared most of losing my chosen family forever.

Finally, we were ready for what would be the first round of our In Vitro Fertilization (IVF) adventure. IVF protocol may look different for every woman. It was medically recommended I do mini-IVF due to my medical history. Mini-IVF includes a ten-day medication protocol, as opposed to the traditional thirty days. I was started on Clomid, an oral fertility medication, often used as the first step on the traditional infertility journey for most women. During the first part of the round, I would go to the hospital for blood work. A few days into the round, I began injecting Follistim into my abdomen every other day (pending test results). Follistim is a hormone that regulates ovulation and the growth and development of eggs. I would report to the hospital at least every other day (again, pending test results) for blood work and a vaginal ultrasound. The blood work measured my blood levels to ensure that I would not ovulate too soon before the egg retrieval. The vaginal ultrasound monitored the follicles: how many were developing and how big they were getting. It was always a fine balance between allowing them to mature, but not let them get too mature. Once things were looking good, meaning the follicles were of a certain size and maturity, I started Lupron (a medication used in IVF protocol to recruit and develop follicles) injections, also in the abdomen, and the egg retrieval was scheduled a couple of days later.

My stimulation did not ever go as planned or according to the original timeline. My egg retrieval was moved up due to hyperstimulation, my body responding too well to the drugs. Upon the day of egg retrieval, we reported to the hospital very early for Chad to give his semen sample (in a cold stark room, without internet access, at 5:30am is nothing short of asking a man for a miracle). I was then started on light IV anesthetics. I was unconscious during the egg retrieval itself, which lasted about thirty minutes. During the egg retrieval, doctors used a vaginal ultrasound and needle to drain each follicle, hoping for an egg that could then be extracted. The viable eggs were sent to the lab to meet up with Chad's sperm. They had dirty martinis, made small talk, and united in the hopes than one would form a healthy embryo, which would then be frozen five days later.

Michelle began her medication once the healthy embryos were frozen. Michelle's protocol was much longer than my ten days; the goal of my protocol was to stimulate the eggs and time ovulation with the retrieval, her protocol's goal was to get her uterine lining nice and thick, and ready to accept our embryos. Michelle was also on Lupron injections, along with Estrodial pills and patches; basically, a lot of estrogen storming her system at once. She then started the progesterone injections a few days prior to the embryo transfers. Progesterone injections are not easy; big needles and the medication is actually administered within a thick oil. They are painful injections in the butt. She would also get ultrasounds to check how well her uterine lining was thickening up.

Both Michelle and I had had minimal side effects and frustrations during this round of IVF. We talked often about our anxieties and excitements and planned for Ben and Michelle's trip to Saint Louis for the transfer. I was very uncomfortable during my minimal stimulation IVF protocol due to medical complications with my back. I lived in sundresses because my abdomen had become so swollen with growing follicles, putting more and more pressure on my lower back. This round for retrieval was pretty standard, although it was unpredictable that I responded so well to the drugs and came close to being hyperstimulated. Hyperstimulation is when the ovaries become overly swollen and sore and the increased estrogen and progesterone levels can create bloating and digestion difficulties. When you read the message boards and get the numbers and statistic low downs from the clinics, you realize how unsuccessful IVF really can be. You continue to feel hopeful and excited but nervous and scared…and angry, cynical, etc. all at the same time, but to be in the hell of IVF and get the numbers yourself, is something none of the message boards or the doctors can prepare you for. I had fifteen follicles develop, the doctors retrieved seven eggs, two of which were not viable and of the remaining five, only two grew into healthy embryos, which were then frozen while Michelle started her medication back in Indianapolis. Our clinic recommended that we transfer both embryos, especially since we had planned for this to be our only round. Chad and I, Ben and Michelle all agreed.

In December, Ben and Michelle left Nathan and Lyla with friends and family and came to Saint Louis for the transfer. It was a quick trip, but one that felt right all the way around. We continued to bond with

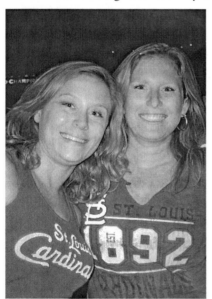

one another, and again realized how similar Michelle and I are. We both have red hair, we both love dancing, we both have the same sense of humor, and we both put others ahead of ourselves and tend to be overly sensitive. But it was also the weird and quirky parts of our personality that were eerily similar, silly things like how we both eat the bottom half of cupcakes and the chocolate sides off of candy bars first.

Michelle and I, more alike than different.

Her numbers looked good. Her uterine lining was nice and thick and the transfer went very well. Michelle let me be present in the operating room during the transfer. I would have never guessed that just thirty seconds of my life could mean so much. Looking into Michelle's eyes, both of ours full of tears of joy and sheer terror, I knew with all my heart that I was supposed to have her in my life forever. It was like looking in the mirror, but also like looking at the reflection of who you know you are meant to be all at the same time. This was going to work! We were all going to live happily ever after, just like all the IVF clinics promise.

After the transfer, we went back to our house and vegged out the rest of the day. We hoped and prayed that the next two weeks would pass quickly. We also hoped Bosco, our rescue Chihuahua, knew something we didn't. Bosco didn't leave Michelle's side the day of the transfer, almost as if he had a sense that something very important was happening. Looking for hopeful confirmation, we had faith that his keen sense with children and babies was spot on.

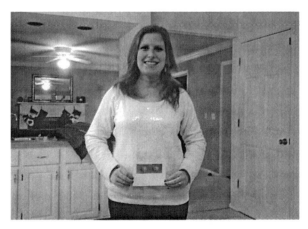

More than just our internet oven.

There are a lot of things the IVF clinics don't tell you before the journey or throughout. The first is how difficult that two-week wait is, especially in the situation of surrogacy. The two-week wait is the time between the day of the embryo transfer and the first pregnancy blood test. During this time, Michelle and I stumbled to find our balance of not talking too much or in too much detail about everything little thing she felt. It was torture! Our two-week wait also happened to fall right over the Christmas holiday. Since we had been so open with our friends and family about our journey, we were able to go home and share with them our amazing story thus far. We also had pictures of the embryos to show off. They looked so strong and healthy in the picture, everyone was sure it had worked. We had already been through so much... we knew we deserved this. Our two-week wait ended on December 28, 2011, when we got the phone call that stopped our world.

Chad and I are one of those balanced couples. Chad is extremely laid back and even keeled, while I feel every emotion in the book, usually to the extreme. Especially prior to IVF, one could have said we were very opposite. Just look at our career choices, Chad the accountant and Justine the mental health therapist. My training and education, even my personality is to feel emotion, and to feel every side of everything, sometimes all at the same time. He is stoic, numbers based, and so relaxed. There would be times throughout our marriage, especially prior to the IVF journey, where I would look at Chad and ask him if he had ANY emotion on a particular subject! Through our years at these emotional ends of the spectrum, Chad has always been great at knowing what I need. We hadn't necessarily planned to be together for the pregnancy test results phone call, but he knew we needed to be, so he showed up at the office I was a subleasing at the end of our workdays and we called the clinic results line. As soon as you hear the voice on the other side of the line, you know in your gut that it is not good news. Yet, there is still that glimmer of hope shining deep inside, convincing you that everything has worked out okay.

The hope that has built over the last two weeks of waiting, the positive thinking that propelled you through the last two weeks. You keep telling yourself, "We have one of the best doctors, we have a young healthy surrogate who has achieved two easy pregnancies (one of them not even planned!), and we are both young and healthy, we take care of ourselves and the real clincher...we deserve this... of course this will work!" Then you hear the voice say those words.... "We are so sorry, she is not pregnant." As it turned out, there was nothing in her system at all. Our embryos, our babies, didn't even try to implant...

There are no words for how crushing it felt. The wind knocked out of me. I was sick to my stomach. My anger was rising, and all I could see was the utter pain and sadness in my husband's eyes. How could we be so delusional? How could we have been so positive it worked? Why was this happening? Hadn't I already paid enough of my crap ass, bad luck karma in life? I honestly don't remember what happened right after we hung up with the clinic. I think we sent Michelle a text to tell her I would call her tomorrow, and I'm sure we called our parents to let them know. Then we cried. I sobbed for the next three days at least. I canceled my clients for the rest of the week and wallowed.

For the first time in my life, talking it out with my loved ones was not helpful, and many times left me feeling a ton worse. I knew there was nothing they could say to make it better and that anything they said would probably make it worse, but that didn't make it sting any less. You get the whole gamut of reactions. I heard a lot of "I'm so sorry." One of my best friends tried to find the silver lining and suggested that maybe this was God's way of showing us we should just try to have our own baby. God love her, she meant well, but this shut me down so quickly! It's not like we hadn't thought of that $15,000, lots of pain and suffering and terrible hormones ago! I had some loved ones that just listened, and said nothing at all. Some cried with me. Some offered to bring crap food and several bottles of wine. Some that would try to make us laugh, including one friend who stated that if we decided to adopt she'd prefer if we adopted a white baby. And it worked, in that split second

I laughed in shock at the political incorrectness of her sentiment, and I knew she loved me so much and was just trying to take away some of the pain. They tried. I love them all even more for how much they tried, but ultimately, there is nothing that can help in that depth of grief, except, "I'm so sorry, I'm here." I tried to distract myself some by running errands, but inevitably someone would call to check on me and I'd start crying all over again. At one point, I called Chad (who had to go into work that day) sobbing. When he asked where I was, I had to admit I was in the parking lot of the vacuum store, I couldn't drive home, and little kids were now starting to point at the scary lady crying in her car.

We said we were only going to do one round, we had a healthy surrogate and a great doctor and very limited finances, but the loss of the two babies was more than we could take. We knew that if we were going to try again, we had to try soon. It's impossible to be immune to the IVF message that every day counts, that each day my eggs were dying and we were losing our chance. It was Kelly, one of my friends and colleagues, who helped us put it into perspective. She said something to the effect of, "In the midst of losing two babies and grieving them, you must make the life altering decision of what you are going to do next. But you have to ask yourselves; in twenty years, are you going to be able to look at each other and be okay with the fact that you tried something that had only a less than fifty percent chance of working and you only tried it one time?" We applied for the loan the next day and got on the IVF clinic's schedule for an April transfer (four months away).

The journey of IVF must push forward and quickly, almost never giving you a chance to take a breath and fully grieve the losses you are suffering. We pushed forward by prepping both Michelle and I for another round of medication. One of my closest friends, who had gone through her own, very long battle with infertility, always told me how every round is different. She couldn't have been more right. Round two, for both Michelle and I, was much more difficult. Harder in the sense that we all knew this was really it, if this didn't work, we would be finished. None of us knew what finished would look like. However, round two was also much more difficult because both Michelle and I experienced a lot more of the side effects of the drug regimen; the mood swings, the hot flashes and the weight gain. My weight went to where I've never seen it before. I've never had a high metabolism and always had to at least workout to maintain a healthy body weight, but my body during round two of IVF was raging against me. I felt terrible; I looked like I was in early pregnancy, and no matter what I ate and how much I worked out, the weight kept piling on. Nothing stings worse than being asked if you are pregnant when you just lost two babies, you are starting another round of IVF drugs, and you aren't even capable of carrying the baby yourself. Talk about a major shame spiral…I'm fat, I'm a worthless woman who can't even do what I'm put on earth to do, and even my eggs suck. This shame spiral fueled by all the hormones was the perfect storm.

The mood swings were also super difficult, especially for Chad. I'd suffered with depression since college. My family history of depression was triggered after witnessing a client try to kill another client at the substance abuse clinic I interned at, medication helped me manage it up until that point, but the hormones of IVF turned the managed depression into the ups and downs of what felt like PMS in hell. One night, I remember yelling at Chad, "I hate you and I love you, please just let me storm off and cry by myself!" Once in bed, I texted him, "I'm sorry, I totally realize this is the Clomid crazy train, but I just can't seem to get off! I'm sorry, I love you!" To which he responded, "That damn train ;), I love you."

Since round two was filled with major side effects, it was also the first time I started to experience frustration with the whole process of IVF. I felt the anger and the bitterness start to boil inside of me. Reading stories in the headlines of people "who don't deserve to have kids" would set me off into tirades or crying jags. Hearing the fellow women waiting in the tiny ultrasound waiting room bragging about how many eggs they have frozen already, and this round was just a precaution, I wanted to scream, "SHUT UP YOU STUPID BITCHES! YOU ARE AT LEAST TEN YEARS OLDER THAN ME, YOU ALREADY HAVE CHILDREN! I HAVE NONE, NO EGGS AND THIS IS MY LAST CHANCE!" In classic culmination, my last day in that tiny ultrasound waiting room, a woman decided to paint her fingernails. None of us said anything! I think we were honestly so shocked she was actually doing it, and a little afraid that if we said something we would all explode and tear her to shreds in a Clomid dazed fog. It was on this day we learned that I was hyperstimulating again and we would have to retrieve the eggs sooner than planned. This round, numbers were technically worse, fifteen follicles, two eggs, and only one embryo.

Our second and last round.

Our last chance for a family, would all lie on eight cells of one microscopic embryo.

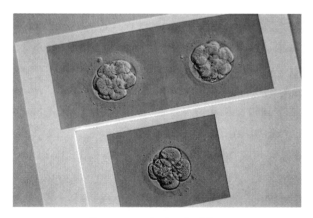

Our never to be babies.

For this round, Ben, Michelle and their kids all came in for their spring break. We had an amazing visit. Chad and I treated them to the attractions of our great city, Saint Louis. We went to the zoo, the City Museum, and bonded as a family. It was wonderful! Michelle's sister, Rachael, came in the day of the transfer to help with the kids while we were at the hospital. More chosen family! We ate dinner the night before, and our fortune cookie read "You are about to embark on a most delightful journey." Of course, the only way to interpret the fortune at this time was this was it: we were going to have a baby!

The transfer was difficult. They changed the medical protocol and wouldn't let Michelle pee at all. The wait felt like forever. For the first time in this whole process, she asked Chad and I to leave the tiny private waiting room. I knew she felt awful. She was embarrassed, in pain, worried and feeling every emotion in the book. I just tried to be there for her. Once she calmed down, Chad and I rejoined her and Ben in the tiny waiting room, we took our picture of her and I in our sterile garb and laughed at the tape on her nose ring. But the anxiety was palpable. Our doctor promised her he would get her to relax and that she didn't need the Valium. Michelle, again, allowed me in the operating room with her. Again, we looked into each other's eyes through tears, the same and yet new, tears of joy, tears of fear, tears of nothing but abandon of authentic vulnerability. In less than one minute, our last chance at having children entered into the infamous two-week wait. That afternoon, Michelle and I spent the day laying around talking and laughing. Again, Bosco wouldn't leave her side, actually laying on her belly for the remainder of the day. We watched episodes of our favorite show, *New Girl,* and we told stories of our journey so far. Michelle adding exactly how our doctor got her to relax while she was on the table that day, by caressing her butt and saying, "just relax, there you go, just relax." Considering what our doctor looks like, and that we've all seen the picture of him in a tuxedo amongst real life penguins, it is an image and a memory that will always make us laugh.

Our chosen family was solidified this trip. My house felt empty and too quiet when they left. The next two weeks were pure agony.

The phone call came on April 16, 2012. Michelle was not pregnant.

After your first failed round of IVF, you definitely prep yourself for devastating news. We had felt so blindsided and stupid for assuming it would work the first time, I think Chad and I both thought about this round in a different way: not expecting it to work but of course hoping. Hoping with that constant cautious hopefulness you seem to have to master throughout the journey of infertility and IVF. Again, we heard the words, "I'm so sorry, she isn't pregnant." I remember having this moment of looking into Chad's eyes, of seeing the sadness and pain of the last year but also the joy and the love that had grown, both between us and between us and our now chosen family; Ben, Michelle, Nathan and Lyla. It was a huge loss, but one that I trusted, at least somewhere deep inside, because it was, for the first time an answer. Now we know, now we can move forward.

The finality of this loss came with every emotion in the book, sadness, anger, fear, bitterness and frustration. Every single emotion applied to every single thing in our lives. What did this mean now? How are we supposed to go on? And one of the biggest questions, in our hearts and I know on a lot of our loved ones minds, where did this leave us with Ben and Michelle? But I knew it was just a part of our story.

Michelle and I continued to stay in contact on the phone and through Facebook. In July, Chad and I went to visit. It was the first time we saw them after the transfer didn't work. Memories flooded through me as we pulled into their quaint little town. The last time we had been in Indianapolis was for our first meeting. How long ago that all seemed. But, I also knew it had all unfolded exactly as it should. We had an awesome visit. We spent great quality time with Nathan and Lyla, and again, built our family on top of the foundation the journey of IVF had created for us. We loved these people. Michelle was meant to come into my life and I knew she would never not be in my life.

In the next couple of months, I struggled some with the thought of Michelle becoming a surrogate for another couple. I knew she was considering finding another couple to be their surrogate, and I couldn't help but be jealous and maybe even a little hurt; even though I knew this was a calling and dream of hers. What if it works for someone else? What if they find another family and forget about us? I was once again thrust into that place I experience over and over as a therapist. I get to feel all sides of every story and feel empathy for everyone involved. We talked about it, just as we talked about everything, and I trusted that she would always be open and honest with me, and I knew my fears were unfounded. She was my family, and no one would ever come in between that. Little did I know, our bond would be threatened, and not in the way any of us would ever expect.

I could hear it in her voice immediately; Michelle called and said she had to tell me something. She was dreading it, but couldn't keep it from me any longer. "I'm pregnant…by accident." I could hear the fear and confusion in her voice and my immediate response was, "Are you okay? How are you feeling? How are you doing with it?" She immediately went into mommy mode and told me all about how other people felt about it, how upset they were with her, etc. I again asked her, "But wait, are you okay? How are YOU?" In that moment, I knew my friend needed me. I couldn't even begin to fathom how I felt about it on the phone in that moment, so I knew I just needed to be there for her. We hung up and I called Chad, who was supposed to work late that day. "Michelle is pregnant, by accident." His response, "I'm coming home, right now."

There are no other words or any other way to feel than total, utter, dumbfounded disbelief. How could this be? We paid over $30,000 (and are still paying back the loan) to get her pregnant. We both put our bodies, our relationships, our lives at stake and in jeopardy with hormones and drugs to get her pregnant. She already had her two kids, they were done with their family… and yet there she was, pregnant, by accident with their third child. I was angry, hurt, sad, and once again felt bitch slapped in the face by life. It was difficult to talk with her at first, hard to hear how difficult it was for all of them to adjust to the fact that they were going to have another baby. Difficult to hear that she was struggling to feel excited about it. Difficult to balance between my role as the friend, who's also a therapist, and who I am - the infertile woman who she was supposed to have a baby for.

But ultimately, our relationship means more to me than holding onto hurt and anger.

I made sure I was there for her. I made sure to validate everything she was feeling and going through. Because it had to be hard, she had a kid in middle school and a kindergartner, now she had a baby on the way. That's a huge adjustment for anyone. I wanted to make sure she knew I wasn't going anywhere no matter what. I had a couple of close friends and family members say to me that maybe this was a sign they weren't supposed to be in our lives. I know they said it out of love and concern, knowing how impossible it would be for all of us to see her be pregnant and have a baby that wasn't ours. But I just knew, we would all get through this, this wouldn't have happened if it wasn't supposed to. I also knew how difficult it is for others to truly understand our relationship and what we had been through. They are our chosen family, literally, and now we were going to face another test of what our destined family could survive.

In December, fairly early on in the pregnancy, they all came to visit us in Saint Louis. I knew it might be difficult, but I also knew I needed to see them, especially before she started to show her pregnancy. More so, I knew they needed to see us. I knew they needed to see that we were okay. That we weren't angry with them, that we still loved them and that we weren't going anywhere. Michelle mentioned that she would love for us to come out when the baby was born, and I was honest in saying that we would just have to see what was going on and how I was feeling. Deep down, I knew I probably couldn't be quite that strong.

Tipton was born in June of 2013. He was such a perfectly beautiful and healthy baby boy. For the first month or so of Tipton's life, I had my own type of postpartum depression. I did not admit this to Michelle at the time, only to Chad and few close friends. Every time I would get a text picture or Michelle would post a picture of Tipton on Facebook, I would torture myself by looking at his features, "convincing" myself he looked like us. He had blondish hair, he had Chad's ears…could he be ours, is that possible? I knew it was scientifically impossible, but my life thus far, had felt like the scientifically impossible made possible. I confessed my thoughts to my friend who had been through IVF, because I knew that the crazy irrational part of my brain would trust her, and that there was no way possible that Tipton was actually our child. My temporary insanity lasted about a month. I knew in my heart of heart's he wasn't our child. I also knew I didn't want him to be our child. That would have been an awful scenario! It was just a defense I developed to get me through the culmination of losing our three babies and of seeing my friend have her own bundle of joy when she was "supposed" to have ours. She was supposed to have my baby, it was supposed to be my baby shower, my new joy, but instead it was meant for her.

The first time Michelle brought Tipton to visit, I was definitely nervous. What would it feel like to have this new baby in our house, to see him after so many months and a pregnancy that wasn't ours like we had all planned? I knew it would be okay, but I also had everyone else showing concern for the visit. As always, it just fit. I loved getting to spend time with Michelle and Tipton, just the two of them. It is always like no time passes between Michelle and I. To hold and smile at this beautiful baby boy, who isn't mine but who I know is an extension of this love between us and our chosen family, I felt complete and like everything was exactly as it was meant to be.

I have no doubt that Michelle and I will always be a part of each other's families. Her family is my family in so many ways. I will always be here for Nathan, Lyla, and Tipton, and I have no doubt that we have so many more incredible memories to make with our chosen family. When I look into Michelle's eyes and I hear her voice, I am reminded of that powerful moment when we looked into each other's eyes during the first transfer. Never could we have imagined what was ahead for us. Never could we have imagined we would have the story we have, or the one that has yet to be written. Never could we have imagined the ups and downs we've survived through together. And never could I have imagined I would find myself, my home and my destined chosen family all from a woman I met online.

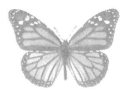

Chapter 2

Setting a
Surgical Foundation

I've danced my entire life. I love dance, even to this day, I do it every single day. However, it is in a much different way than I had hoped growing up. My dream was to attend the University of Iowa on a dance scholarship. The time and money my parents spent carting me, at the end of my dance career, forty minutes each way, two to three times each week to class was the signature of a family who believed in my talent and my love of the sport. In the early spring of 1992, when I was eleven years old, it started getting more difficult. My stamina was waning and my body began to hurt and ache in ways I had never felt before. Pain unlike anyone should feel, especially at that age.

I would spend the car rides home in tears, both out of pain but also of frustration in not being able to dance the way I knew I was destined to. The pain had just become too much.

In total, my family spent a year and half going to doctor after doctor searching for answers as to why my hips and back hurt so badly at such a young age. You couldn't get me to stop dancing and since no one ever said to stop, I danced through the pain. I could barely walk at this point. My first misdiagnosis came from a very well known and brilliant hospital where they put me through some of the most painful tests I've ever experienced. After putting cameras into my hip joints, they diagnosed me with Conversion Hysteria. The doctors actually accused my mom of forcing me to dance and that my mind was making up the pain. They claimed there was nothing physically wrong with me and they sent me to a sports psychologist. That moment, at the young age of thirteen, was the most invalidated and misunderstood I've ever felt. My parents were heartbroken. Little could we have known that this misdiagnosis would single handedly change the course of my entire professional life. It was the first chance I've had of many, at redefining myself and my dreams.

You lose one dream, you figure out a different one.

The sports psychologist taught me how to visualize the pain outside my body so I could continue to do the thing I loved most, dance. She validated me in that she didn't support the Conversion Hysteria diagnosis but still sent us home with no answers. I was still in major pain but now armed with the skill of visualizing the pain outside of me. She was my first glimpse into the world of psychology. I had no way of knowing what the future held, but I knew that I felt drawn to her and what she did. As we headed home to Iowa answerless, and still in major pain, I knew in my heart of hearts that I'd found some spark of light to guide me forward.

The next, and thank God brief, misdiagnosis was a possible tumor on my spine or pelvis. Numerous bone scans and MRIs and the first of a torturous two week wait later, it was confirmed that I did not have a tumor or cancer. But yet again, we had no answers. Again, no one was able to provide me with any validation of what I was going through, both of my pain and of the bleak world of knowing something isn't right but not having anyone able to find what was wrong.

The misdiagnosis that would ultimately save me from my own body was that of fibromyalgia. Fibromyalgia back in the early 90's was not well researched or documented, especially for a thirteen year old. I was treated with pressure point massage and lots of medication. At one point, I was taking about ten pills a day to manage the pain. Amazingly, we had a fibromyalgia specialist pass through the Quad Cities and she was willing to look over my records. It took forever; there were hundreds of charts, notes, x-rays and other tests for her to go through. My clearest memory is of her coming out to the waiting room and asking if anyone had ever said the medical terms spondylolsis or spondylolisthesis to us. We'd never heard these terms, even though my charts and notes were riddled with them. Bottom line, she saw a fracture (spondylolsis) on L5 with a grade 4 slippage (spondylolisthesis) on a year old x-ray from a chiropractor. She referred us to a specialist who happened to be a dancer in her past life. Another set of bones scans determined there were actually two fractures on the last vertebra, L5, and they were from an old injury. This doctor then referred us to Dr. Stewart Weinstein at the University of Iowa Hospitals.

Dr. Stewart Weinstein was the nicest doctor I had come into contact with yet, and he was our angel, our kind hearted, always smiling, dazzling white haired doctor with the super-hot resident. The hours our family spent sitting in the waiting rooms of the University Clinics were countless. We packed books, homework, games and food, because inevitably we'd be there no less than four to six hours each time for me to see all the specialists. Through the boredom, we also shared many hours of laughter in these waiting rooms. My sister, Kristy, always the comedian; as much as she drove me crazy, was a huge piece to our survival as a family through the long, boring and difficult hours waiting in hospitals. We were also constantly reminded of how blessed we were. I was almost always the most able-bodied patient Dr. Weinstein saw, many of his patients suffering with debilitating cerebral palsy or other spine disorders. After all the waiting, both in Dr. Weinstein's waiting rooms and the entire last year and a half, we finally had our answer. I had fractured my spine. It was quite possibly the scariest answer I could have received, but it was an answer nonetheless. Finally, some sort of validation. We were told that my injury, two cracks on L5, is a common injury for dancers and football players. Often times it is found sooner and can be cured by bed rest and medications. Since the injury was so old, there was too much scar tissue surrounding the fracture and my back surgery was scheduled for two weeks later, just as I should have been starting my freshman year of high school.

On August 25, 1994, Dr. Weinstein took bone from my own hip and fused L5 to S1. For those of you that don't know, your spine is made up of thirty vertebrae. L5 is the last of the lumbar vertebrae, right above your tailbone, and S1 is the first vertebra of your sacrum. The point of the fusion was to fuse the fractures on L5, regain proper spine alignment and eliminate my chronic pain. It was a long surgery. My most poignant memory is that of being wheeled back to my room after recovery and seeing my Aunt Kelly's face full of sheer terror, sadness and love. The first three days I was in and out of consciousness due to excruciating pain and the morphine pump. I spent the next eight days in the hospital, lying almost naked in a hospital bed, rolled like a log to check drains, and being asked if I had to poop yet. Being asked if you have to poop is something no thirteen year old girl should have to endure. Once the drains looked good, I was put into a full body cast. Dr. Weinstein and his super-hot resident casted me into a purple body cast while I held myself up with handles suspended from the ceiling and a bar across my lower back. The cast went from my chin to my hip on one leg and to my knee on the other leg. My options were to lie down or stand, while holding up a thirty pound plaster body cast, for the next six months. Dr. Weinstein sent me to Occupational Therapy to get my body upright. They put me on a tilt table for a few hours slowly getting me upright,

Being wrapped in the body cast.

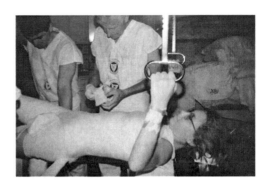

Left: Full body cast for six months.

Below: Part of the body cast and an old picture in the wheelchair.

since I had been laying down flat for the last seven days. It was in there that I learned how to sort of walk with crutches and was shown different tools to help me put on socks and go to the bathroom. Then we were sent home, in a laid out wheel chair, to fend for ourselves.

There's nothing more effective at making you thankful for your small, and usually too nosey, town than suffering a life altering tragedy. Our local America Legion donated a hospital bed to put in our living room since my bedroom was on the second floor. The local Lion's Club built a massive handicap ramp outside our front door, so I could be wheeled in and out of the house, especially to get to my follow up appointments. People I'd never met sent get-well cards, including handmade cards from whole classes at my school. The local newspaper did several stories on me and my family. I had teachers come to my house during their free periods to teach me my lessons; my English teacher also videotaped her classes for me. The generosity of this small town and the school system is why we were able to get through this immensely difficult time. I didn't fall behind in school at all, and was even able to maintain my nearly perfect GPA.

For six months, I was in a body cast, lying down or standing/semi walking with crutches. I spent my days hanging out with my nurse, Shelley, cross stitching, and watching *Days of Our Lives*. I had great friends who came over, forced me out of the house, and made me laugh. I had friends who left, not being able to handle seeing me in that much pain or not sure of what to say. But, how much can we really expect of freshman in high school? I also had friends step up who I never would have imagined sitting next to me throughout the journey. I have cringe worthy memories of how bad my haircut was and how the only thing I could wear was men's boxer shorts and huge t-shirts and overalls. Luckily, overalls were "in" at the time, this was the 90's, but still difficult for a fourteen year old to feel confident in, especially considering the extra thirty pounds of plaster cast I was toting around. I remember trying to figure out how to wash my hair in the hospital blow up sink and my family realizing that just picking me up like a board onto the kitchen counter was much more effective. I remember how hard we laughed, when I had to trust my little sister to shave my legs. My little sister, who was always taller than me, the same sister who tortured me growing up by pinning me down and farting in my face or spitting over my face and sucking it back in, and now I had to trust her to shave my legs?!?! I remember how resourceful my parents were, always rigging something up to try to make our lives just a little bit easier. They built an ergonomic handle for people to push my wheelchair around instead of having to bend over to do so. They built ramps with tracks up to our minivan in order to get my wheelchair into the van to transport me the forty minutes to follow up doctor's appointments, then tarp strapped me in for "seat belt safety". The most brilliant fix was for the most asked about dilemma of being in a body cast… How did you go to the bathroom? Without much dignity, but hey, everyone poops right? My dad rigged up a raised seat with part of it cut out for the portion of my leg cast and attached handles to the bathroom walls and someone would have to hold me while I lay across the toilet seat. This was as a hysterical an image as you may imagine, but also the place where I have had some of my most honest, heartfelt and uncontrollable laughs. Because sometimes, all we can do in times of terrible trauma and tragedy, is laugh and take our minds off the pain. I believe this was an integral part of my growing resilience. Besides, what other choice did I really have?

Eventually, things were looking good and I was able to get the leg portion of the cast cut off. I slowly went back to school. We survived it. I was released to normal activity, but I was not ready to return to dance. The next three years passed like any typical small town high school girl's life would; boyfriends, student council, friends, and good grades. Then I attempted to join the track team, and things just didn't feel right. An MRI confirmed my fusion did not cure or heal as well as they had hoped. For the first time in my life, I learned what it meant to be in the unlucky percentile. I was in the 10% of spinal fusions that didn't take, and I would need a repeat surgery.

The June before my senior year of high school, Dr. Weinstein fused L5 to S1 again. This time I was put into a body brace for six months. The brace still came from my chin down to my hip on one leg and to my knee on the other leg, locking my left hip joint. I was much more able-bodied in the brace versus the thirty pound cast, so healing seemed to go faster this round. However, we had some complications this time, including our insurance refusing to pay for a stay at home nurse, so my parents paid my best friend Kelly C. to stay with me. Nothing brings two sixteen year old girls closer than one having to hold the other on the toilet while she goes poop while also making fun of her the whole time. Once again, some of my most hysterical laughs of my life were during those moments, where I chose to be vulnerable and human and not choose shame because I knew that wouldn't help me survive it. On the other hand, I'm not sure I really had much of a choice. One of my favorite memories is when Kelly insisted that we go for a "walk" and get out of the house. As I was ambling down the ramp with my crutches, one of the crutches slipped off the ramp, which meant, since I couldn't bend at the waist, I timbered down like a tree right onto my face. I clearly remember that moment of sheer terror; oh my God, can I move my toes? Then I just laughed, because that had to have been quite a sight to see. This and the fact that all I could hear was Kelly running back to the house and then back to me screaming, "Oh my God, are you alright? Help she fell!" I know some of Kelly's favorite memories are of the laughs we had washing my hair, shaving my legs, going to the bathroom, really just every day moments. Kelly is a major brick portion of my surgical foundation, she played a huge role in why I didn't turn over and die and instead chose to thrive through it all. We have been through hell and back, literally and together.

A few weeks after my second surgery, I was sent to the hospital for pain in my upper back. At first they thought I had dislocated a rib from an awkward movement in the body brace. After hours in the ER and the most painful oxygen blood test ever, a chest x-ray finally showed I had pneumonia and a lot fluid in my right lung. I was admitted, put on IV antibiotics and my right lung eventually had to be drained. Very scary, considering I had to be taken out of the body brace, also because it was my mom's hospital duty day that day and she doesn't do needles, let alone huge needles and tubes to drain a lung! She did amazingly and her voice helped to keep me conscious during the procedure.

Healing moved pretty quickly after the pneumonia episode. I returned to school much faster with the body brace because it was easier to walk/hobble around in. So much easier in fact, that I had to carry an allen wrench with me to tighten the locked hip joint because I was moving around so well. I felt so good. This was it, I was healed; and from the darkness emerged a new me with a new dream.

Finally, during the second semester of my senior year I was healthy, earning good grades, student body president and getting ready to leave for college. During my back surgeries, I was the only one from my graduating class to apply and accept attendance to an out of state school. I honestly never thought I would get into Truman State University, I just figured I would attend University of Iowa or University of Northern Iowa like everyone else. Even after all the years of support from my amazing small town, I was ready to start over and didn't want to be known as the dancer who couldn't dance anymore or as the girl in the body cast. I knew this was my destiny, I knew I needed to leave the warm embrace and safety of my small town.

What I now know, twenty years and hard therapeutic processing later, is that those two surgeries and that year in the body cast left me unhappy, pissed off and without a voice. I was literally trapped in a body cast for a year of my high school experience. Yes, I had amazing help and support, but knowing what I know now, I was also really alone. As much support and help I had during that time, it was sympathy. It was pity. I was surrounded by people who felt sorry for me when all I really wanted and needed was empathy. Someone to say, man this really sucks, I'm sorry. The pity, the sympathy, simply left me feeling even more alone, and that coupled with the cast left me a shell of my spirited self. A shell that would only be completely filled back up after losing three babies and choosing recovery.

So my parents moved me to Kirksville, Missouri to attend Truman State University in the fall of 1998. We had the worst first day ever. The residence hall didn't have my name at all, it was hotter than Hell, and none of the furniture was easy to put together. As mom and dad were packing up our minivan, getting ready to make the drive back to Iowa, I stood on the curb. I started crying, and begged them to take me back saying, "I changed my mind, I'll go to Iowa instead." As always, my parents pushed when I needed it, just a little, and did what had to be one of the hardest things they'd ever had to do as parents; they left me standing on that curb.

College was four years of finding myself, learning a ton, and having some of the best times of my life. I met amazing, lifelong friends, got my heart broken too many times (mostly because I kept choosing the wrong guys, like most girls in college), was able to return to dancing on the dance teams, and I found my true love: my new passion, Psychology.

I was a psych major from the very beginning and I loved every second of it. I started working in the field right away, the summer after my freshman year, I interned at the local adult substance abuse center. This is where I came into contact with every type of person possible and experienced firsthand working with every disorder people struggle with, including learning more about the disease of addiction. This is where I learned that boundaries are important with clients, but they also have to be balanced with true passion and care for what you do and for their recoveries. I made many mistakes and witnessed too much to understand back then.

It was during this time that my own depression was triggered. I'd grown up always knowing depression was in my family history on both sides, even to the point of several suicide attempts. I'm sure there was a part of me that believed I would never suffer with it, both because my sister struggled some in high school and because I had survived a huge trauma, twice, and it still wasn't triggered. However, as we say in the field, genetics loads the gun but environment pulls the trigger. While working at the substance abuse clinic my junior year in college, I was the only staff monitoring clients when a client attacked, to kill, another client. He had relapsed on methamphetamines and gone off his schizophrenia medication. Then and there, my trigger was pulled. I began having night terrors. I was able to smell and taste in these vivid nightmares, and had a hard time figuring out whether or not I was in a dream or real life. My mood fell and depression set in. I was put on Remeron, which helped tremendously with sleeping, and my mood began to lift. This was again, a time in my life where true friends came through. People come in and out of our lives for reasons we may never fully understand. I lost some friends and gained new ones, and was once again surprised at who shined in helping me get through the darkness of depression.

I graduated early from Truman due to my internship and stayed in town to work as a Community Support Worker while my friends were finishing up their semesters. I also applied to graduate schools and hoped to gain residency in Missouri as to not pay out-of-state tuition again. My time in Kirksville, Missouri, a big city to me, only continued to build my foundation, now the foundation of my profession that is ultimately most of who I am in so many ways.

Moving to the "really big" city of Saint Louis for graduate school was a step I never would have thought I was brave enough to make.

But, I knew that in order to start my career, I had to earn the advanced degree. Most of my friends from Truman were back in Saint Louis following graduation, so I had a support network already in place. I loved Saint Louis, and still do, and I loved graduate school. I worked full time throughout graduate school and continued to fall more and more in love with psychology, human nature and connection. I bought my first home on my own, and then unexpectedly, and when I definitely did not have the time, I met Chad, which is typically right when life brings your person into the light of your life.

Chad was one of a couple of single guys invited to a float trip with a few single girls through some mutual friends of ours who were already married. It was a day of drinking and floating down the river, full of laughter, reminiscent of college fun. The entire day, I was sure he was interested in my other friend. Then night fell, a flaming marshmallow was accidently flung on my lap, and the rest as they say, is history. After the float trip, he didn't call until late the third night after asking for my number, and I let him know that I noticed. We had an amazing first date and we spent the next year and half dating. During this time, I sometimes faltered in opening up my independent self and life to a partner, but Chad's self-possessed stoicism was already present in the building of our foundation.

We were married in Iowa on October 28, 2006; the night after our beloved St. Louis Cardinals won the World Series. We had no doubts, ever, and no inkling of the difficulties that would lie ahead for us. It was an amazing day. A wonderful day, with one major hope missing, it was assumed it would always just be us: kids weren't possible.

I'd spent most of my teenage and college years never allowing myself to want to be a mother. Rather than get my hopes up of having my own children, I actually stated out loud that I didn't want kids and faced the wrath that comes with speaking out against doing what women are supposed to do and what we are supposed to want. Throughout

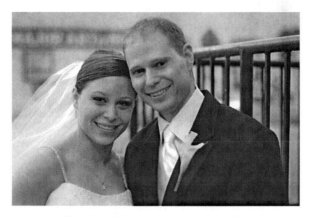

Chad and I on our wedding day.

the years of medical treatments I received in high school, I received hundreds of x-rays, MRIs and a plethora of other tests. All on the region of my lower back and hips, all unshielded. Each time I was asked by the x-ray technician, "Is there any chance you could be pregnant?" The answer always being no and the follow up question always being, "You understand we can't shield your ovaries for this film?" But what choice did we really have? I was thirteen years old, in pain, at times barely able to walk, and no one could tell me what was wrong with me. Take the x-ray, fry my ovaries, I just want to be a normal teenager. Looking back, I know I never realized the power of those tests or the chances I was taking. I have no doubt they play a part in my non-mother status in life. Not only would I never be able to choose to carry a pregnancy, both medically recommended and through my willingness, but I am sure they are the very reason surrogacy did not work for us. My eggs just aren't my babies, at least in this life on earth.

When I'm asked how I survived living a year of my life in a body cast, my response is never earth shattering. I didn't have much of a choice, so I chose to be resilient. Although my back surgeries are the very reason we sought out IVF treatment to conceive our family, they were also the foundation set beneath me that helped me to survive and thrive after

IVF. I tell my back surgery story to explain my big scar or why it's hard for me to stand for long periods of time or because someone has asked about my past. I tell it hopefully to inspire others who think they can't keep fighting or they can't change their life. But I also tell it for myself: to remind myself of how strong I am, how much love and help there is in this world, and simply because it makes a damn good story.

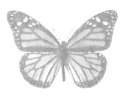

Chapter 3

Owning Adoption

e stopped the IVF treatments before we got the baby. We stopped the drugs, the hormones, the painful and expensive procedures all before we got the intended result. We stopped before we got what we paid for and what we wanted and hoped for. We knew our IVF journey needed to end. We knew it wasn't going to work. For our health, emotional and physical well-being we had to stop. We also chose to not take the most common, and what most think, is the most natural next step after failed IVF. We are not choosing adoption. My truth means I didn't get to have my own children from IVF and adoption isn't right for my family. Owning those two decisions, however, is another feat all in itself.

One of the first questions many of us are asked when meeting someone new is, "Do you have kids?" I respond every time with, "We tried, but can't." I will own this response every single time. I don't say it for pity. I say it because it is my truth, my story, and if I shy away from it, all that results is shame. So I own it, whether or not it makes you uncomfortable. I almost always get a flustered, "I'm so sorry," in response. Then more often than not, the person I'm speaking to blurts out, "Well, why don't you just adopt?"

Why don't we just adopt?

These simple words are often spoken as a way to help and "fix" my pain. They are said because my loved ones believe I'd be an amazing mother and they just want me to have that joy. They are said because we are uncomfortable with pain and sadness and we will say anything to make it go away fast. I know they are spoken out of love and are well meant, but they tend to cut like a knife. At least they used to. These five words feel invalidating to the journey I've been through. I suffered through and survived IVF. I've lost three babies and three lifelong dreams. Suggesting that adoption can take away that pain and replace those three babies feels downright hurtful, like a dig right to my soul. These simple words also minimize the journey of adoption, suggesting it's really as easy and uncomplicated as just stopping by the store to pick up a baby. In reality the journey of adoption includes tens of thousands more dollars, more pain and loss, and usually years before your family is truly and securely complete. Even though I know these words are spoken out of love and curiosity, I also know they are spoken because it is the journey of so many families, especially following IVF failure. They are spoken because it seems to be the natural next step to failed IVF. But I also know, with all my soul, they are not the words of my story. When asked so simply, it feels like they shine the shame light onto my story. The shame light, that until now, I have allowed to silence me.

Chad and I knew throughout the IVF journey that adoption was not for us. I suppose you can never be sure how you will feel when IVF fails, but it was something we'd always been on the same page about. Chad has been very open and honest in saying that it has never been an option for him. For myself, being a therapist, I feel like I almost know too much about Attachment Disorders. I've also been on every side of adoption throughout my career; the mother who has had to live with giving up her child, the mother struggling with her adopted child, and the adopted child who never feels like they know who they are or where they belong. I know there are millions of amazing adoption stories out there, and very healthy ones at that. But I also know myself, and my family with Chad, and our path has never included adoption. It has been scary to admit this to ourselves at times, but even scarier to own it to the outside world of our friends, family and even strangers. Everyone has an opinion, and loves to offer a quick fix.

It is beyond terrifying to openly admit that adoption isn't for us. I am fearful of being judged and misunderstood. I'm scared people will think I never really wanted children since I'm not willing to go the length and adopt. I'm scared people will think I'm a bad person, who doesn't want to give love and "save" a child through adoption. I'm scared of the judgment, that since I am a therapist, I am REALLY supposed to want to adopt. Ultimately, I'm scared of what every other human being on earth is scared of. I am scared of being judged. I am scared of being misunderstood. What it truly comes down to is that I'm scared of not being known, seen and loved. Even though this may be an inherent fear for all of us, when we live our truth, our path in life, and we live it authentically, it is going to include a lot of these fears. However, I can choose whether or not it makes me close up and hide from my story, allowing the floodlight of shame to drown me. Or, I can work with this fear, embrace it, and really own myself again. I can learn to trust that the bravery it takes to state that adoption isn't for me, owning that limitation, is better and healthier than not listening to my soul.

The journey of Ever Upward, of redefining myself after IVF, has been two fold as I've chosen two not so popular choices; stopping treatments and not adopting. I stopped IVF treatments before they worked and I'm not adopting. The message being sold by IVF clinics is one of just keep trying, we recommend another round, and we believe this will work for you. Throughout the journey we not only felt rushed to make decisions but also never validated by our team. It wasn't until our second egg retrieval that our doctor told us he was, of course, recommending another round, especially considering we only had two eggs retrieved, but he understood that we may need to be done, both financially and emotionally. This hopeful, "it will work message," is also being portrayed in the media time and time again, especially by celebrities. It is amazing that celebrities and the media are beginning to talk more about infertility and IVF, but the message being delivered is dangerous and creates even more shame for us in the real world. This message of "just keep trying," "never give up," and "it will work" is hardly ever delivered with the accuracy of how painful and expensive IVF is. This message delivered by celebrities with endless resources, especially in comparison to the average, everyday American like Chad and I, an accountant and self-employed mental health therapist, both with significant school debt left. The fact is that IVF doesn't always work. Quite frankly, a majority of the time it doesn't work, some research states that it actually fails 70% of the time! We need to start this conversation and stop shaming people into round after round of dangerous hormones and medical procedures and tens of thousands of dollars. This shame only leads to emotional turmoil and many times it results in marital distress. It is okay to stop; it is okay to say no more and to accept what is. However, that is only a decision that each family can make for themselves.

When we decided that we were finished with IVF after the second failed round of treatment, many of our loved ones, and even strangers would tell us to just try again. In these moments, I never passed up the opportunity to do what I believe I do best, educate. People need to realize the physical pain and risk that go into these treatments. That, bottom line, I have no idea what the hormones or Clomid could do to my body in ten or twenty years time. But, I also needed to speak out about how much IVF costs, especially with a surrogate. Each round of medication and procedures cost about $15,000, plus Michelle's compensation. Insurance does not pay for these treatments, and I'm honestly torn as to whether or not they should, as I see both sides. But as someone who is still making a monthly payment towards the loan we took out for our second round, it is the part of the story that needs to be spoken. After much anger and resentment, I now know we make those monthly payments not for nothing, but because I've changed my entire life following this journey for the better. So even though that extra $20,000 was for another chance at babies, it really was for another chance at this life; this life as a happier and healthier, better person.

Saying no to adoption following IVF is a very foreign concept to many people, including our family. Shortly after our last failed round of IVF, we were approached by some of our close family about adopting a distant relative's unborn child. Chad got the phone call and I could tell right away that he didn't want to tell me what it was about, but knew he had no choice. Again, I completely understand these family members asked us out of love and hope. Love and hope for everyone involved. But it was especially crushing and confusing to me. It felt like our journey and losses were being invalidated, again. It was hurtful because it felt like no one took into consideration how much this may set me back emotionally. I had finally started to get back on my feet and feel like myself again. It was also absurd, considering the relative in question was barely pregnant and hadn't even gone to the doctor yet. It would have been such a crazy, messy, and complicated situation and one that I'm not sure would have ever been okay. In my heart, I knew this wasn't our baby. I knew I didn't want to adopt. But to try to explain to Chad how it all made me feel was so difficult. Potentially, a healthy newborn baby, who may even look a lot like us, was available to us. I would be denying myself if I didn't admit that there was this part of me that had always dreamt of opening up the door to find a healthy baby on my doorstep needing a good loving home. I knew this was an irrational desire, and yet was one I'd had for a long time, considering I'd always known I'd never carry my own child. At one point, Chad looked at me and asked, "Are you upset because you think this is our baby?" I knew that wasn't the reason, I was upset because I felt like no one understood what we had just been through. I felt minimized and invalidated. I was upset because I didn't sign up for the adoption journey, and there we were forced into it, smacked right upside the head in the face of major loss and still grieving. No one, including Chad, may ever understand how hurt, and frankly re-traumatizing, the whole situation felt to me. Knowing it was from this place of everyone wanting to just take away our pain, give us the joy of children, and make it better didn't make it any easier for me to swallow.

Nevertheless, what I am now learning to understand is that it is okay to feel loss and pain. Sure it isn't the most pleasant part, but it is an important part of our stories. Without pain, without loss, we would not get the experience of joy and love, which means we'd never be growing.

"Why don't you just adopt?" is no longer a string of hurtful words that spark anger inside of me. I am able to embrace the intent of love they come from. I am able to own my life in sharing my story. I will speak my truth, the truth of saying enough is enough and that no, I will not adopt. I will speak my truth because if I do shame cannot exist. And without the shame of this journey, I am more and more able to embrace it all and own it. Ending IVF treatments and knowing adoption isn't your path, also means finality…for everyone.

A huge part of this ongoing journey has been working to understand and support our loved ones and their loss in this journey that comes with our decision to stop treatments and not adopt. My friends will never get to see me parent or get to love on my children as much as I love loving on theirs. My sister will never get to feel the joy I feel being an aunt to her children. My parents will never be grandparents to our children, who would be closer to them geographically than my sister's children. My in-laws, most likely, will never be grandparents. Much of my hurt and healing is very much shared, if not paralleled with our parents' pain and suffering. I know they've suffered these same lost dreams; they lost three grandbabies in our journey too. I also know they will spend the rest of their lives mourning these lost dreams and adjusting to feeling like they are not "normal" to others their age because they aren't grandparents. The loss and emptiness leftover after IVF has led to this sense of not belonging, both for myself and for our parents.

Now, as an adult woman without children, I'm struggling, for the first time in my life, with a sense of not belonging. By the classic and most widely accepted definition of a woman my age, I will never fit in. I am not a mother. I am constantly reminded of this; in the congregation full of families, in the group of moms discussing feeding or soccer schedules, in the childfree by choice group (some of which don't even necessarily like kids) or on Facebook walls which are filled with pictures of birthdays, the first day of school and the holiday Elf on a Shelf fun. I don't fit in, and if I hold onto the losses, the hurt and the shame too much or too long, I definitely won't ever belong.

But this choice is mine. If I can own my choices and therefore my whole story, I will always belong. Embracing my fears, accepting my losses and owning my story means I have the power. The power to be happy. The power to educate. The power to make a difference. The power to stop proving that I'm okay. Stop just proving that it's okay to say no to IVF. Stop just proving that it's okay to not adopt. Stop just proving that you can be happy without children even though you wanted them. Stop just proving that you can be whole and happy, even if your life doesn't look the way you had hoped or envisioned it. To stop just proving all of this, in order to truly own it.

During this part of my journey I've come to realize that perhaps I've almost been born too late. If I were 20-40 years older, we perhaps would have tried to have kids but to no avail. No one would ask about it openly. If we didn't adopt, people wouldn't publicly shame us. Back then it was shameful to be childless, and you didn't talk about it publicly. You would sadly whisper under your breath, "Oh, they never were able to have children. It's just the two of them." There was no Clomid or IVF. If you couldn't have kids, you just didn't, and you either adopted or figured out your happiness just the two of you. Now, we have medical miracles and the endless options of treatments and routes to having children. People are more comfortable talking about it, which is a great start but in some ways has resulted in pushing shame into the light, rather than owning it to lessen it. As loving as the intention may be in someone's inquisitiveness of why we stopped treatments or why we aren't adopting, it often times is more about doing what is considered the norm, which then makes it feel like something I am doing wrong, and leaves me feeling different, alone and judged. However, these feelings are mine, I must own them in order to heal and redefine, to find my version of my story.

And, in my version, we have adopted, or at least our version of adoption. Less than a week after our last negative pregnancy test, Chad and I rescued our version of twins, thirteen week old Chihuahua Miniature Pinscher puppies, litter mate sisters. We knew our older dog, Maddie, was not doing well and her health would continue to fade to the point of us having to make another impossible decision in our lives, to put her down. I got Maddie as a puppy when I was single and had just moved to the big city of Saint Louis. She was my first true love, my first furry child. And when Chad came into my life we only fell in love even more. Maddie was, unfortunately, a puppy mill puppy and was not aging well at all. She would often need to be hospitalized due to chronic pancreatitis. When she was hospitalized our other dog, Bosco, would depressively wander the house looking for her, wallowing in the saddest way possible. We knew Bosco would make a terrible only child. We had always planned to transition from two dogs to three, then back to two when Maddie started not doing well, which we envisioned sometime in the not too distant future. But then, when we lost the last baby in the second and final round of IVF and our dreams of having human children were yanked away from us in a thirty second phone call, we knew it was time.

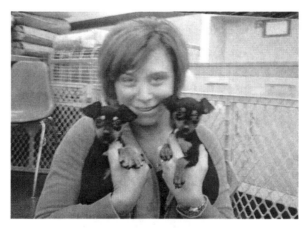

Adoption day.

Chad found the girls at a rescue in downtown Saint Louis. He came home saying they were adorable and that we should go look at them the next day before someone else adopted them. So that weekend we went into the city to a somewhat run down, but brightly painted, pink rescue shelter. The girls were still there, sister puppies. The rescue worker said we had to meet them both at the same time as they were only thirteen weeks old and had never been apart. He claimed we wouldn't be able to get a feeling for their personalities if we met them separately. Genius sales and marketing ploy, or the truth… definitely doesn't matter now.

In walks the kindest and most soft spoken black man with a head full of beautiful braids halfway down his back with a tiny puppy in each hand, three and a half pounds tiny. They were adorable and hysterical and I knew we were taking them both home. We played and we laughed and Chad and I looked at each other in disbelief…we're going to have four dogs for a while. Sitting in that not so great smelling, pink animal shelter with Chad and these two tiny puppies, I felt authentic joy, for the first time since starting IVF. I called my parents to let them know that we were actually bringing home two puppies. I will never forget my dad's words and he will probably never know how much they meant to me. He said, "You're grieving. You're not crazy, of course you're adopting both of them. You guys finally deserve some happiness!"

The girls were named Gretchen and Grace. Gretchen seemed so demure and peaceful that day that I insisted on switching her name to Gracie. And par for the course in our family, we renamed Grace to

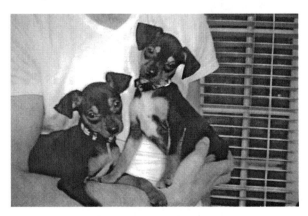

Our version of twins.

be Gertie, which is a Seinfeld reference like Bosco. We headed home to introduce our twin girls to their siblings. Having two puppies was definitely a test of our patience but one that IVF had probably prepared us for more than we could have acknowledged then. In addition to lots of love, therapy and a lot of support from our loved ones, having two puppies was also the best cure for getting us through the grieving process. There simply is nothing better, in my opinion, than puppy love and play, let alone times two! Watching them grow, learn and play provided us with pure love and joy. To this day, those two girls make me laugh every single day and warm my heart so much. They have completed our family.

As crazy as everyone thought we were for having four dogs, we knew it was the right decision for our family at the time. Maddie's chronic pancreatitis was getting worse, and then she tore her meniscus in her back leg. Very quickly we watched as her soul left her body and we knew it was time for us to make the second impossible decision of our marriage. It was time to say goodbye and put her down. Outside of deciding to stop IVF and accept our lives without children, making the decision to put Maddie down was the most difficult decision we've had to make, but, then again, it felt right.

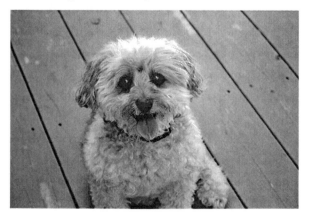

Our Maddie.

The last day of Maddie's life was a great one, for her and our family. My parents came down to celebrate her. She got the first real bone of her life and spent the day chewing (with her terrible and barely there teeth) and being loved on more than she probably cared for. She also spent the day with Gracie constantly by her side, just nudging closer and closer, whining to be close to her. Gracie is so easy to read, it was like she was saying "Come on, I just want to love you and be with you before you go." Little did we know it at that time, but Gracie's constant attention on Maddie that day definitely resulted in Maddie's spirit moving into Gracie. Since that day, Gracie has been anything but graceful and just like Maddie in all the weirdest quirkiest ways.

The next day, Chad, my parents and I took Maddie in to say goodbye. My dad was not even able to enter the office, all of us were sobbing. They started her IV and the doctor explained what would happen once he administered the shot. Everyone then left the room for Chad and I to say goodbye and have a last moment with her. In true Maddie fashion, she pulled out her IV. Saying goodbye to Maddie will probably be the hardest thing I will ever have to do in my life. She saw me through some very difficult times. She was Chad's first true pet love. She was our first child, furry sure, but our first nonetheless. But, we knew it was time to let her go. The staff was amazing that day. The nurse and doctor administered the shot and left us with her body. My body has only been ravaged by heart stopping, gut-wrenching sobs like that once before, when we lost the first two babies.

We petted her, loved on her, prayed over her and said goodbye. That was the only time Chad has ever allowed tears to actually flow down his face in front of me. I don't know how long we stayed with her. Through our tears, of course, eventually came laughter, as has always been the case in my life. Hugging her and kissing her, a stench rose into the stale air of the hot, tiny room. The doctor had explained that an animal will often times pass gas once the medication takes effect, as it relaxes everything.

Chad and I both smelled it, it was just awful. I asked Chad to check, make sure that she didn't poop, because it smelled awful. Taking one for the team, for our family, Chad confirmed we were in the clear, just gas. Later that night, he told me that I will owe him forever for that, as it was like looking at a huge empty tunnel, since everything in her body had relaxed with the medication. In fitting fashion, we were a team faltering and stumbling our way through our loss with our laughter and our love.

In less than a year's time, I'd suffered more loss than my blessed life has ever suffered before. Losing Maddie in the wake of ending IVF was a devastating blow. Someone put it perfectly about losing Maddie. When you lose a person in your life, there is always some sort of baggage or emotional hurt, but when you lose a dog you are losing something that has provided you with true unconditional joyful love 100% of the time. He said it will always be one of the biggest, if not the biggest, loss of your entire life. He's right; I think of Maddie every single day still and say her name out loud at least once a day. This is, however, also due to the fact that Gracie is Maddie reincarnated. It is uncanny and sometimes just downright eerie how similar Gracie is to Maddie. The way she plays. The way she growls at everything, including when she is happy and loving on you. The way she whines and whines and whines at her siblings until they will give up their chewy for her. The way she could eat all day long if we let her. The way she tilts her head from side to side when you talk to her. The way she loves on everyone, all of the time. Best of all, the way she just loves. She is a daily reminder of the joy that can be found in every moment of every day, even in the darkest of hours.

Sitting with anger, sadness, depression and bitterness is okay. I think it is part of everyone's journey, especially after suffering major loss, trauma or tragedy. And man, did I sit in it for a while. Losing Maddie was the permission my depression needed to come in and help. The depression came back; it helped me to cope and try to heal. But eventually, it moves from sitting with the unpleasant emotions of anger, sadness, depression and bitterness to sitting in it. It no longer is a coping skill or defense mechanism that is helping us to survive but becomes the very thing that is holding us back from our hope and healing. I began to struggle with this shift. I was now knowingly struggling with what I help my clients with every day in session. I was sitting in the shit, no longer sitting with it. I now was in it and choosing to stay in it. I couldn't cry any more. I couldn't scream how unfair it was any louder. I couldn't feel so much anger at the people who were having babies but didn't "deserve" them. I couldn't be sad anymore. I had to help myself.

Life decided to define my rock bottom for me in losing Maddie. It was time to take that first giant step out of rock bottom and into recovery, back into life.

One Google search later, of infertility therapists in Saint Louis, led me to my therapist Shellie. When she called me back to ask what I needed to work on, I gave her a shortened version of my hellish story, and stated that, "Bottom line, I just lost my dog and it seems to have sent me over the edge." We scheduled to meet the next day, and thus began my decision to choose change and the year of work that has changed my entire life for the better, the work that is my Ever Upward.

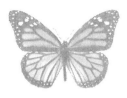

Chapter 4

Choosing Change

Disclaimer: I chose to change many pieces of my life in choosing recovery after infertility. This chapter is not meant to be a how-to or even a sure fire answer to others on what steps they need to take to change their own lives. Rather, this is simply an explanation of how I did it. Take what applies to you, or what you think you'd like to try, and leave the rest. We all have to simply find the strategies that work for us, because only then will we choose the change and do the work to continue it.

I had tried therapy several years ago but never really felt a connection. Truthfully, as a therapist myself I should have been in therapy much sooner. A good therapist will utilize his or her resources, colleagues, and therapist friends, but a great therapist will see his or her own therapist. I knew I had one hell of a fight in front of me and I knew I needed to start the work, to put one foot in front of the other, and I needed someone to walk alongside me through it. I didn't need that person to help me to make decisions about the IVF process as they were already made. I didn't need a place to vent about how terrible IVF was. I just needed a place to learn how to navigate my new reality, accept what is and find myself again. I needed therapy to help me implement the new me and to help me follow through on choosing change, choosing recovery and choosing myself.

In the fall of 2012, I started to make major changes in my life. I will probably never be sure of what worked the best or if it truly was a combination of everything. In the fall alone, I changed my lifestyle (food and exercise), changed my medication regimen and started therapy. I continue these all today, along with several other pieces I've added along the way.

I've always had to work to maintain my weight and health. I considered my metabolism slow and accepted that as long as I worked out, my weight would stay healthy. After the hormones and other drugs of IVF my metabolism felt like it stopped, especially considering the IVF medications also added at least twenty-five pounds to my very short frame. I've been both blessed and lucky to never struggle with poor body image, despite growing up a dancer, but for the first time in my life, I was super uncomfortable in my body. The weight didn't feel good, I hated the way I looked and I just didn't have the energy I had before IVF. It was even more frustrating because I had gained all this weight to no avail. I didn't have the happy bouncy baby to show for it. Eating healthy and doing my normal workouts didn't seem to be cutting it anymore.

After sharing my frustrations with my friend and officemate, Kelly, she told me about the Blood Type Diet in *Eat Right For Your Type* by Dr. Peter D'Adamo. She said it had always worked for her, especially when she needed to get back to her healthy self after having her two sons. She also said that some of our dietitian friends, who specialized in eating disorders, might not like the food plan due to thinking it was too restrictive but that it had always worked for her. She told me to read the book and see if it felt right for me. I downloaded it that day. Dr. D'Adamo's research has found that each blood type digests foods differently. Reading his work, I felt it instantly click for me. If Chad is a blood type O, and I am a blood type A and we both eat a banana, why would we think we digest them in the exact same way? Our blood types help to determine how much acid is in our systems, how much mucus we produce, etc. This all effects how we digest food. I felt the fit and moved forward. I set the deadline for the beginning of September to start and commit to this complete lifestyle change.

Ironically, the very cause of having to find this new lifestyle was also the place who had my blood type. I called the IVF clinic the next day and found out that I was a type A. Dr. D'Adamo puts food into three categories for each blood type: Beneficials, Neutrals and Avoids. You can eat as much as you like of the Beneficials, these foods are like medicine to your body. Eat Neutral foods within balance, they aren't particularly beneficial but aren't harmful to the system either. Finally, limit if not cut out entirely the Avoid foods, as they do not interact well with your system. What this method meant for this 'Iowa corn fed girl, born and bred on meat and potatoes' was a complete overhaul. Dr. D'Adamo's recommendations for blood type A meant no red meat, no potatoes, no gluten and no dairy. He recommends you follow the plan about 80-90% of the time for optimal benefits, which felt like a great balance for me.

I had one week left to enjoy some of my favorite foods including one of my favorite meals; a ribeye steak, potatoes and corn, and man did I start the blood type diet feeling like shit! Chad supported me by eating 100% type A at home, even though he is a type O. Not that he has much of a choice; since I am the cook in our family, type A had dibs! It took me a couple of months to feel comfortable going out to eat at restaurants, but now know I can always find something. Starting the blood type diet has been nothing short of miraculous for my life. Within the first two weeks of living this way, I was sleeping better and had more energy. The weight started to come down at a steady and healthy pace. My digestion finally felt normal. I was no longer starving on a dime and felt more satisfied with the foods I was choosing, even though I didn't need to eat as much. The single biggest difference though, was no heartburn. I thought I would always have Tums in my nightstand drawer, I just thought this was something genetic. Before the blood type diet I would average at least six Tums a day, however, after finally choosing to change my food, I haven't had heartburn since, unless I have a free day with food and eat whatever I want.

I have learned a major lesson in balance by sticking to the blood type diet. When it comes to food and exercise, very rarely is it healthy for anyone to do something 100% of the time. More often than that, it is often times just unrealistic. For the most part, I have cut out my big Avoid foods but will definitely still enjoy the breadbasket occasionally. And I don't think there will ever be a day that I don't miss ribeye steaks. I always beg Chad to order one when we go out, just so I can have that one succulent bite. Following the blood type diet 80-90% of the time has allowed me this balance and freedom. Following it consistently has also helped me to become much more in tune with my body. I've learned which foods are okay to splurge on and which ones just are not. The occasional gluten usually just means my weight will be a little high, but the occasional white potato means that no one will want to be around me and I will feel miserable. The blood type diet may not work for everyone and I know there is a ton of research discrediting it, however it has worked for me and I highly recommend at least trying it.

Reading Dr. D'Adamo's research, I also learned that he recommends certain types of exercise for each blood type. Typically blood type A's tend to be highly anxious people; I was not surprised by this at all. For the management of stress and also the biological changes that happen when we experience stress, he recommends exercises such as walking, hiking, swimming and yoga for blood type A's. I had spent my entire adult life doing weights and hard-core cardio in an attempt to manage my weight. I had even achieved mild success with P90X a few years before starting IVF. I've never been one to do anything half ass, so along with changing my diet, I also changed my workouts.

I try to walk the dogs for twenty to thirty minutes at least a few times a week, although the unpredictable St. Louis weather can make this difficult some of the time. I practice yoga once or twice a week, weight train using my own body weight twice a week, and usually throw in a high intensity interval training or a Tabata workout twice a week. In reality, I probably workout about twenty to thirty minutes, five to six times a week, mostly due to my schedule and some very early mornings. Additionally, I make sure to do some random dancing, by myself, every day. I no longer dread working out, I actually enjoy it. I have used Pinterest in the way I think it was intended to be used. Not to make you feel like you aren't enough, but just to give you more ideas. I love finding random workouts on Pinterest, that way I never get bored. Using these workouts makes working out at home and within less than thirty minutes very doable. But, if you find that you just can't get motivated to workout at home, then make sure you join a gym, or get a workout buddy, and get that workout in.

Changing my lifestyle, food and exercise wise, led to the IVF weight and then some finally coming off. My skin is more manageable. My anxiety is lower. I am sleeping better. My overall health and wellbeing is much improved. It wasn't an easy change and did require discipline. I started to feel so much better so quickly, that I was able to keep my motivation up to continue. However, the food and exercise overhaul, is not the only big player in choosing to change my life and fighting for my recovery.

Once I started therapy and doing the work I needed to get back on my feet, I realized that my medications were no longer working for me. In a lot of ways, it was like the hormones of IVF had reset my brain. However, I must admit I was also just over the weight gain that Remeron causes. I was put on the Remeron in college for help with depression and night terrors. The major side effect of Remeron is around ten pounds of weight. My sleep had always been more important to me than the weight. Wellbutrin was added a year later to try to counter the weight gain from Remeron. I had been on this same cocktail for 11 years. It had always seemed to work, and once when my mail-in prescription order was accidentally canceled, I realized how much I actually needed the medication. But after IVF, it seemed as if everything had been tripped in my body and in my mind. I had also found ALPHA-STIM®, and it was finally the permission I needed to finally try to go off the medications.

I stumbled across ALPHA-STIM® in a way I wasn't supposed to, in relation to not yet published research. I had started the process of becoming certified in ALPHA-STIM® in order to use it with my clients, but had yet to consider it for my own personal use. ALPHA-STIM® (cranial electrotherapy stimulation) is a prescription medical device indicated for the treatment of anxiety, insomnia and depression. Safe enough for home use, ALPHA-STIM® delivers a signal very close to the body's own electrical system via ear clips. This low current allows the client to come out of a fight or flight response, and helps the brain to enter into an alpha state. Clients become very relaxed in the alpha state, similar to the effects of meditation. ALPHA-STIM® is best used as an adjunct to medication and/or counseling and may help a client progress faster during counseling. Research indicates the majority of clients see benefits, with minimal to no side effects.

During the certification process, I was able to witness one of the most powerful sessions of my entire career. I had been working with Angie[1]

---

1   Name has been changed for privacy.

for three years. She had always struggled with rigidity, perfectionism and debilitating anxiety and had been on medication for five years with minimal benefit. The first time I put ALPHA-STIM® on her, she reported she had not felt that relaxed since she was a child. For the first time in three years, she actually sat back on my couch, completely relaxed and at peace. I have been certified in ALPHA-STIM® for over a year. I have seen it change the lives of many of my clients. It has also gotten many of them off all of their antidepression and antianxiety medications. I am also one of ALPHA-STIM's® success stories.

I started using ALPHA-STIM® in the late fall of 2012. I was able to get off Remeron within about six weeks and Wellbutrin within three months, under the care of my psychiatrist of course. ALPHA-STIM® has changed my life dramatically. My sleep is sound and my anxiety and depression are much more manageable. With an over 90% success rate with minimal, if any, side effects; I think it can be a viable option for many. But, as I tell my clients, it has not been a cure all. I have used my lifestyle change with food and exercise, with the addition of the ALPHA-STIM® to give me the motivation, and on some days, the strength, to do the really hard work of recovery; self-care.

So much of our lives could be helped simply by changing our self care. How we eat, sleep, move and cope. Often times, I am able to help my clients so quickly because we first look at and conquer their self care problems. So many times I am asked, isn't self care selfish? After fourteen years in the field, I can honestly say that many of the people I see are simply not selfish enough. I think selfishness has gotten a bad rap. I am not asking my clients, or myself, to be self-centered or arrogant but to simply be selfish enough to take care of themselves first. Because if we don't take care of ourselves first, there will be no one to take care of our loved ones.

When educating clients on changing their eating habits, I will of course share with them what I do with the blood type diet. But more importantly, I help them to find what will work for them. Often times this is just helping them to find balance, variety and moderation with food. I also help my clients work on their relationship with food. Yes, it is social and can be emotional in our culture, however we need to do the thought work to change to thinking about food as our medicine and fuel. I also help them think of different activities for movement and figure out a way to find the same balance, variety and moderation with their exercise routine. Something, I've also struggled with. A couple of summers ago I tried to train to run a 5K with a friend. I was never really that excited about doing my training schedule, so one Sunday Chad offered to run with me. Just the sight alone, is worth a good laugh, Chad, a 6' 2"former decathlete, running (really walking) alongside myself, a 5' former dancer. God bless him, he tried to encourage me as I was cursing up a storm. About a quarter-mile in, he finally looked down at me and said, "Why are you doing this, you hate running! Don't you always tell your clients to do exercise they like!" I looked up at Chad and said, "Why AM I doing this? I fucking hate running!" I am proud to say I haven't run since. I would so much rather do a video at home, dance like a crazy person or take a mindful brisk walk than run. The point is to find something you at least like, but hopefully love to do, for your daily movement or exercise. You're definitely more likely to keep it up if you enjoy it.

ALPHA-STIM® has helped to improve my sleep, but I've also worked very hard on my sleep hygiene, or sleep routine. My clients always stare at me with a look of confusion when I ask what their sleep hygiene is, because inevitably at least 75% of the people who come into my office to help improve their lives, aren't sleeping well. By sleep hygiene, I mean your nighttime routine. Our parents worked very hard when we were younger to implement a consistent nighttime routine. We had a bath, read a story, maybe said some prayers, and then it was time for sleep. We did the same thing in the same order every single night.

We prepped our brains to slow down and get ready for rest. The need for this nighttime routine, I believe, only increases in our adult lives. Our demanding and constantly overstimulating adult lives makes our brains go into overdrive. To think we can simply lie down in our bed without slowing down and get a good night's rest is futile.

Working on a nighttime routine can be frustrating and time consuming, but I promise it is totally worth it. Chad always teases that my nighttime routine takes forty-five minutes, which is only a slight exaggeration, but it works. I fall asleep quickly and sleep throughout the night without disturbing dreams and best of all, I feel rested in the morning. To find what works best for you, simply take some of these ideas and try a few at a time. The key then, is to find which order to do them in. Once you find something that works well, you repeat it every night, every single night. Following a consistent nighttime routine can definitely improve your sleep. Some ideas to get you started

- Writing/journaling
  - o Write about your day
  - o Write the best and worst (peaks and valleys) parts of your day
  - o Write 1-5 things you are thankful for – make sure they are different gratitudes each day. This will help you to be thankful for even the small things.
    - ◊ There are days I am thankful for something huge: a great moment with a client, clarity in my writing, etc.
    - ◊ There are days I am thankful for the simpler things: a pillow to lay my head on, my car is running safely, etc.
  - o Write when you felt your Native Genius™ that day – when did you feel your magic, when did you feel you were living your purpose or calling that day. I learned about Native

Genius™ from Kristen Wheeler at a conference. To find more information, check out her website at http://www. kristenwheeler.com/.

- Coloring
  - o Yes, coloring!
  - o Either in a traditional coloring book
  - o Or, my favorite, mandalas (circles of different designs from the Hindu and Buddhist worlds, often time representing peace, Zen, etc.).
- Reading
  - o An actual book
  - o If you must read on a tablet or phone, make sure it is on the night setting (dark background) as the light is stimulating to the brain. When our eyes detect dusk, they send a signal to our brain to release melatonin, which makes us drowsy. Using technology before bed, with bright lights, prevents melatonin from being released.
  - o Meditative books such as a devotional or daily meditation. My favorite is *Comfortable with Uncertainty: 108 Teachings on Cultivating Fearlessness and Compassion* by Pema Chödrön.
- Yoga
  - o Some light nighttime yoga (I like to find videos on Pinterest, but there are plenty of resources you can use.)
  - o Simple stretching exercises
- Deep breathing
  - o Using guided meditation (download an app or search on YouTube or Pinterest)
  - o Progressive muscle relaxation
    - ◊ Start tensing each section of your body starting at the bottom with your feet.

◊ Tense up that section of your body, take a breath and then let go.

◊ Repeat as you move up your entire body, focusing on each major muscle group at a time.

◊ End with tensing everything together, take a breath and let go.

o Count breaths (only up to four or so, stay away from concentrating too much on the numbers).

◊ Imagine light and relaxation coming into your body on the inhale and stress exiting your body as you exhale.

Doing a few wind-down activities, every night, in the same order will help settle your body and mind down and prep you for sleep. I have found my night-time routine essential in getting off sleep medication and improving the quality of sleep I get every night. Now if I could just head to bed earlier, since it takes me at least thirty minutes to get ready for sleep!

Along with changing my food, exercise and sleep habits, I have worked tremendously hard on my emotional health and coping skills. The most helpful resource for me in this part of my journey has been the work of Brené Brown, especially her book *The Gifts of Imperfection*. I believe her research on shame and vulnerability will change our world. I am so thankful for her work; it has helped me not only to change myself, but also to help my clients immensely. I have been able to take some of her recommendations and combine them with my own life and style to change my daily life. The year after IVF was spent working my ass off to change and become a healthier and happier person. It has been a journey of hard work, but the kind of hard work that feels so good that I haven't minded it all that much. I have learned that I simply have to make the time to do this work. I do believe we all have this time, so many of us just choose not to find it. The longer I am on this journey of self-improvement, the more I have come to realize that unless people are doing this work, I don't think they are living the most fulfilled and happy life they could be. We must practice happy to be happy.

This emotional coping and improved wellbeing has included the changes in my food, exercise and sleep I've described above, but it has also included making other major additions to my daily life. These additional changes include dancing and music, creativity, writing and making sure I work on connection, seeking out and working on my relationships, all as recommended through the work of Brené Brown.

Brené Brown writes about dancing in *The Gifts of Imperfection* as a way of connection through the vulnerability it presents for all of us. As I have written, I grew up dancing and would like to remember myself as being pretty good. But, this isn't the kind of dancing I'm referring to. My passion for that kind of dancing is fulfilled through watching professional performances or reality television about dancers. What I'm talking about is that goofy, fun dancing where you can't help but move to the beat and smile, even laughing out loud. Sure, some of us feel the beat more accurately than others, but bottom line I believe we all feel some beat of the music. Play a couple happy songs and just dance! Jump around, kick a random leg, spin and feel the light of joy engulf you and fill your soul. Don't worry about looking stupid, nothing can look all that stupid when you are smiling and joy is literally spilling from you.

Every day, specifically in the morning, I dance. I play my happy, go get them, power songs by artists such as Kelly Clarkson and Katy Perry or Pharrell Williams' Happy website, and jump around like a buffoon. There are some days that this dancing bounce has to be done in the shower or getting ready or in the car because the morning hasn't gone as planned. Nonetheless, dancing and really feeling the music really gets the day started off in a recovery way for me. I've also found that it helps quite a bit to sing at the top of my lungs, whether in the shower, while getting ready or on the way into the office. Belting it out, for me, makes the happiness level soar.

Making music a more prevalent part of my life has been an extra benefit of making dancing a part of my daily life. I have found that my mood can instantly be changed with the blaring of my happy playlist, especially in the morning. I love all music, but have found that music with a message of what I am most drawn to helps me the most. I think making positive music part of daily living can help someone choose to turn their day around in about three minutes!

Brené Brown also discusses the benefits of having creativity in our lives in *The Gifts of Imperfection*. I have lived most of my life never thinking I had a creative bone in my body. I was always envious of artists of any kind, singers, dancers, painters, decorators, etc. I think I've also always felt intimidated, never making things look good enough or doubting my abilities to come up with new ideas. Brené discusses this type of shame in her research a lot, the leftover shame from our "art scars" growing up. What I have found is this battle of never feeling creative enough, or never enough at all for that matter, is twofold. First, I think I had to find something I truly enjoy. Second, I had to let go of making everything look perfect.

So I started where I recommend all of my clients start, especially for the management of anxiety, depression and insomnia: coloring! In the beginning, I recommend and tried the regular, old school coloring. Get out the box of crayons, the smell alone will take you back to simpler times, and the cartoon coloring book and start there! Then let it evolve. Maybe you like painting more or working with colored pencils. Color in traditional children's coloring books if you prefer. I have found that I like coloring mandalas much better as it sparks my true creativity. If I color in the Disney princess coloring books, I use the same colors every time. For example, Ariel's hair will always be red and her seashell bra purple. When coloring mandalas, I get to choose all possible colors. As I have continued to keep coloring in my life, I have found I really like using markers to color mandalas. The mandalas are beautiful and calming, but the markers are crisp and powerful, the perfect all-encompassing combination for my journey of recovery.

Once the creative juices were flowing, I found myself seeking out other projects for creativity. What better place to wander around than your local craft or art store, just walk around the store and feel which aisles pull you to them. I found myself drawn to the stamps and cards. I have always loved sending cards to my loved ones, but this old school gesture can tend to get expensive. So I decided to attempt to make my own. I started in the dollar bins, since I wasn't sure this new hobby of mine would take off. I have found my loved ones love my perfectly imperfect handmade cards from me, so much better than the fancy store bought ones.

My creative heart continues to find other outlets to shine, as I will share in a later chapter, especially in unexpected places. What I can attest to for sure is that having creativity in my life on a regular basis keeps me connected to myself and vulnerable, which are both necessary in staying happy and healthy.

I have always recommended my clients journal or write a little every day, but I fully acknowledge that it is a piece of self care that is very easily pushed to the wayside and forgotten. Writing or journaling every night, as I've written, is beneficial not only for our sleep but also for our wellbeing. I have never considered myself a writer until I knew I had this story to tell. Adding writing to my weekly schedule through my blog, Ever Upward, has helped continue my healing process. Putting myself out there, unguarded and completely honest, has provided me with so much freedom to feel how I feel and to continue my therapeutic work to heal from IVF and improve myself. Writing has always been therapeutic but I think so many of us are intimidated by it that we never try. Get out a pen and paper or open up the laptop and see what comes out. It is not to make a permanent record of everything; it is simply to get it out. Make the difficult things less powerful and the amazing things even more powerful. Keep it to yourself or publish the blog, whatever you feel the pull towards. They are the words of your story, of your heart; follow them wherever they may take you.

Finally, this year of choosing change was supported by the work I have done with my therapist, Shellie. She has been an amazing fit for the work I have needed to not only survive but to thrive after IVF. From the beginning, she was very honest with me about parts of her story, herself suffering through some of the IVF process and also having two children, one of whom is adopted. It has been so helpful to work through everything with someone who knows the struggles of IVF, but also with someone who has chosen a different path through it. I have had to face myself in her office each session, stating out loud the fears I have, the successes and improvements, but also the anger and politically incorrect thoughts and feelings that come with this journey; including the ones I'd never speak out loud, even to my closest friends. She has helped me immensely in navigating how much my life has changed, how much my marriage has changed and how different I am. She continues to believe in my strength to fight to be so. She has been supportive and helpful as my relationships have changed throughout this journey. Her support in helping me to navigate my evolving relationships has been the greatest benefit of starting my therapy with her. She has been that guiding light to shine a different perspective on who I am. Who I am as a friend and family member, and on who I want and need to be.

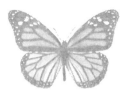

Chapter 5

Evolving Relationships

mbarking on IVF and now choosing a childfree life, I knew everything in my life would change, and I knew it would change completely. Although I was ready to embrace these changes, nothing could have prepared me for how much my relationships would change. Not only would I never have believed which of my relationships have been enhanced for the better throughout this journey, but also I would never ever have guessed which ones have ended or forever changed for the worse because of this journey. Again, this is something that the message boards, blogs and even the IVF clinics did not prepare me for in the least.

I have always worked hard at my relationships. Whether friend or family, I would like to believe I have done a great job of engaging and making sure my loved ones know how much I love them, want to be involved in their lives and assure them that I am here for them, forever and always. I even did my best to keep up with my relationships throughout the IVF journey and continue to do it now, after accepting the losses of IVF. More importantly, I keep up with my relationships after choosing our childfree life, but I never imagined how much more I do.

For many women, the IVF journey can easily isolate them from many, if not all of their relationships. It is filled with so much shame that we place ourselves in a prison created by IVF with shame as our only cellmate. We close ourselves off from loved ones, because they just don't get what we are going through, or we think they don't, or we never even give them the chance to try to understand us. Closing myself off from my loved ones is so incongruent to who I am and how I live my life that I couldn't imagine ever going through my hardest journey any differently. My challenge throughout IVF was to still be myself, ever engaging and loving and communicating, and to see if my loved ones could get it. Because, I knew my loved ones would never get me or what I was going through if I didn't even try to share it with them. So, unlike most women going through IVF, but much more in tune with how I have always lived my life, I lived our IVF journey in the open. I talked about it with my loved ones. I shared with them the dates of everything: the timelines, the waiting games, the medication protocols, the side effects, the fears, and the joys: the everything. I figured that if I shared it all then that meant the more people we had praying and thinking positively for us. I also figured if I shared then I wouldn't feel so alone, with only Chad to rely on and talk things through with. Many women struggle through IVF alone, afraid to reach out for help and ashamed of having to use assisted fertility treatments. I think in this isolation, it is also too easy to get caught up in the message boards and the constant need to Google search every single symptom. This ultimately, makes the journey so easy to become obsessive about, leaves you feeling even more alone and, I believe, can negatively affect your wellbeing, therefore negatively affecting the chance of IVF actually working!

If IVF is going to work, I challenge women to make sure that it isn't the only thing going on in their lives. I believe you must be reading other things on the internet, you must be talking about your job and loves and passions to your partner and loved ones. IVF cannot consume you, because honestly, what if it doesn't work? All the preparation and knowledge you have learned and obsessed about online, isn't going to make it work any quicker or better. And, trust me, it definitely doesn't prepare you for what comes after the losses and the acceptance of what is.

Talking about our journey openly with our loved ones also meant we had to deliver the terrible news when things didn't work. Even though this felt so difficult, and no one could ever say the right thing, again, they were there. They tried to support us. Again, they sent us their thoughts and prayers for healing. They were never easy phone calls or text messages to send out, further solidifying that we were not going to get our own children, that this journey was not meant to work for us. We felt these losses harshly, but we felt them with the love and the support of our loved ones, only because we lived our truth authentically and not on our own, all alone.

Living my truth out loud, even during IVF, for my loved ones to see, increased my chances of being understood and loved through it. Shying away from this would have only meant more stress on our marriage and more shame for me. So I didn't shy away. I owned my story from the very beginning. In doing so, I found that speaking my truth and my story out loud for everyone to hear, if they are open to it, only continues to help my healing and acceptance of my circumstances, and ultimately, helps me to continue to live out one of the biggest parts of who I am, as an educator.

This openness with our loved ones, while helping to keep us grounded, definitely came with an unexpected struggle. Most of my relationships flourished during and after my IVF journey, because of my authentic truth telling and living, but I also have technology to thank. From meeting Michelle through an online surrogacy ad to reconnecting with so many people via Facebook, using technology has enhanced my relationships.

I know there are continued articles and blogs written about how unhealthy social media can be for us, and I have definitely gone through that stage. Before really delving into the work of changing my life after IVF and fighting for my recovery, social media used to be a major source of heartache for me. Like most of us, I would check it first thing when I woke up and last thing before I turned off the lights, not counting the many times I'd check it throughout the day. It took me a little while, with the help of a firm nudge from Chad, to realize that I never walked away from checking my wall feeling better. I was usually sadder, angrier and more frustrated.

Seeing all the pictures of children, the birthday pictures, the snow days, the first days of school, the newborn pictures, etc., the moms getting together, with or without their kids, left me feeling left out. Within this comparison and scarcity mindset, I only had us or our dogs to post about. The comparison definitely got the better of me more times than not. Until, I did a slight detox. I slowly weaned myself off checking my social media walls, limiting myself at first to four times, then three times a day. Moreover, I no longer allowed myself to start and end my day by checking my wall. The moments when I first wake up and the moments right before sleep need to be spent in a connected and mindful place, with myself, so social media was no longer the beginning and the end of my days.

Once I took a step back from social media, it clicked. Finally, there was a sense of connection throughout this social media rather than this itch I have to scratch, or addiction. Through all the changes I had started to make; the reading, writing, exercising, eating better, all the self-care to make myself happier, healthier and whole, I realized that I could use social media for positive purposes too, using it to enhance my life and wellbeing. I would like to think social media was not envisioned to make us feel worse about ourselves: the constant comparing, the competition, the shaming, the arguing, etc. I would like to think it was truly conceived to carry out what we are meant to do as social beings, to connect. So I set out to clean up my friend list. I defriended or hid people who used social media to complain, shame, judge or engage in negativity. I liked pages that were centered on things that are funny, thought provoking or inspiring. I challenged myself to only post and share things that are positive, inspirational or funny.

I also made sure to use social media to actually connect with others. Liking and commenting on other's positive posts. Sending messages of encouragement or *I get it's* or *me too* or congratulations or thoughts of love, support and prayer. It wasn't long before I felt this shift in my participation in social media. I looked forward to checking it instead of feeling as if I had to check it to satisfy my addiction or for outside validation. I learned about myself and others in reading more articles or watching positive videos. Most importantly, I reconnected with my peers, my friends, old and new. I became involved in others' lives, even if just through social media. Frankly, a friend is a friend. Putting effort into these relationships, online and otherwise, was continuing my journey of change. Improving all relationships by putting in the effort, the time and the care meant I was fulfilling more of myself.

Surviving IVF, and now accepting a childfree life, has meant that all of my relationships have changed. The longer I continue to thrive after these losses and live my life, I am learning that all relationships evolve and change, especially following loss, tragedy and heartache. Relationships cannot help but change, grow, evolve, and sometimes even end when we ourselves are changing, growing and evolving so much.

Unfortunately, I had two major relationships change for the worse throughout this journey. One of my closest friends, or at least someone whom I believed to be one of my closest friends, discovered she was pregnant during our first round of IVF. I was so happy for them! Of course, I was a little jealous because they had just started trying, and literally got pregnant their first time of drunken sex. I was happy for them because they were about to begin the journey of becoming parents and happy because it looked like they would escape the awfulness of IVF. The jealousness stemmed from that small part of all of us struggling with IVF that this just doesn't feel fair. Why them and not us?

Lauren[2] was very inclusive with her pregnancy. She asked if I wanted to know how she was feeling throughout the pregnancy, even asking me if I wanted to hear everything she was learning about the baby. For example, how big it was getting or how much her body was changing. I loved it, it was one of the most thoughtful things Lauren had ever done in our friendship. We had always been unlikely friends. I am much more emotional than she is and we both of have very different interests, but we always seemed to have the best times together. Her vulnerability with her pregnancy helped me to feel like we would get to be parents together. Unfortunately, she will probably never know how much her willingness to keep me involved in her pregnancy journey meant to me.

One week before our second (and last) pregnancy test, I threw her baby shower. I was so excited to show them how excited I was for this baby. How much I wanted to be involved in her life forever. I threw an amazing party with a great cake surprise. Everyone had a great time, and I can honestly say it was the perfect way to spend our second two-week wait. It kept me busy and focused on the miracle of family, chosen or not.

---

2   Name has been changed for privacy.

Lauren gave birth to their first daughter about two months after we ended IVF and began the journey of figuring out life without children. I went to the hospital to hear the birthing story and to hold that baby girl with all the love in my heart. I would never get to hold my own, but I knew I would be able to see this little girl grow up and could only hope to be in her life forever. There was never any indication from Lauren that this would never come to be.

Throughout her maternity leave, I felt like I had to beg Lauren to come see her and the baby. I would text over and over, to only get a response about every four times. Looking back, I should have just shown up on her doorstep. I should have just told her how I was feeling. The distance continued to grow between us. I felt pushed aside and forgotten about. Later I learned that she felt like I pushed her away. We had never had the type of friendship in which we talked about feelings and because I let that dictate my actions, I will never for sure know what happened between the two of us. There will always be two sides to the story.

She once told me she felt like I pushed them away because it was too hard for me to be around her and the baby. I know this is not the truth. It felt like the harder I tried to be there and be her friend, the more she pushed me away. I had to stop, I couldn't force her to be my friend, but I had to painfully bring myself to the point of realizing this truth. It was only one of the two times I have gotten very angry about our journey and someone's perception of it. She, I would think of all people, does not get to say I am the sad, childless, infertile, bitter, angry woman. I tried to the point of embarrassment to be in their lives. I loved being around that little girl and them as parents. I love kids. I love my friends who are parents, and more than anything, I treasure having a place in their lives and families.

What I think happened, is that Lauren struggled some with postpartum depression, and as someone with a lot of pride, she couldn't afford to have her emotional, therapist friend know. So she pushed me away and blamed it on my non mother status. We have tried to rekindle once before, and perhaps one day we will, at least I hope so. But, I have no doubt that it would have to be with the agreement to disagree on what happened between us. I am very thankful that my friendship with Lauren seems to be the only one in which her ability to be a mother and mine to not, ended our friendship.

Most of my other friendships only became closer throughout my IVF journey and more so after. Asking for support from my friends was something that was very scary, especially considering most of them were already mothers, but it was worth it. They were all a significant part of our journey and our survival through it.

Throughout IVF and thereafter, I made a conscious effort to make more time for my friendships. I would text, email and call them more. I also made sure to make time for them. Chad and I would try to set dates with their families for the weekends at least once a month. I also made sure to go out to lunch, brunch or dinner with girlfriends on a regular basis, at least once a month hopefully. Making time is the most important part to maintaining and strengthening friendships. This quality time ensured that we would know what was going on in each others' lives. I also made sure to ask about more than the kids. Even my friends who are stay at home moms are more than just moms, even if they struggle to remember that at times. Engaging regularly and putting more time into my friendships, well beyond the general check in, allowed them to flourish and deepen, something that I will forever be grateful to our IVF journey for.

Within this engagement with my friends, I also made sure they knew that I wanted to be involved with their families, even more so now that we were choosing to accept a childfree life. I asked about the kids' events, made sure they knew that we would like to be invited to the concerts and games and parties. I did this for two reasons, admittedly. One, I loved being involved in the kids' lives. I wanted to be a part of their growing up and see their accomplishments. But two, I also didn't want to be left behind.

My friends who are moms are some of my best and most supportive friends, especially on this journey. They are superwomen (even though, a lot of the time, they need to remind themselves that they don't necessarily need to be). They are the hardest working people I know, all working full time, whether in or outside the home. I admire their patience, their unconditional love and their unending strength. There are simply no words for how amazing their love, support and understanding has been for me, throughout this continued IVF journey.

They are also, naturally, the busiest people on earth; raising children, nurturing a marriage and trying to find the time to sleep and do some basic self-care. They have practice two nights a week, games and birthday parties on the weekends and can book up their weekends with other families who have children quickly.

And, sometimes there just isn't time for me, for us, the couple without kids. And that's okay. And I do get it. But, there are times I feel like I want to jump up and down, frantically waving my arms, screaming to them, "But I'm still here!"

I do still have a life I'd like to share with you.

I do still want to hear all about yours.

I do still need you to maintain our friendship.

Ending IVF and living a childfree life could very easily mean I lose my peer group. The crushing blow of not being able to fulfill my dream of motherhood means I have more time; more time for self-care, more time for my marriage, more time for my friendships. I suppose this can be an 'ever upward' of failed IVF and accepting a childfree life. However, it also can feel pretty isolating, as most of my friends, especially my mom friends, don't necessarily have this 'luxury'.

But, it is my job to tell them if I need more. If I am feeling left out, that is all on me. If I need more from my friends, then I need to ask for more, and if they can't give more, at least I know I asked for what I needed. If I am feeling left out, that is truly on me.

I have also learned that there will be times we ask for what we need but our loved ones just aren't able to give it. I have learned this lesson with a close loved one, thankfully the only other relationship that has significantly changed for the worse because of my journey. Throughout our journey, Marie[3] was mildly supportive. She never quite knew how to ask the questions about IVF or how we were doing throughout the process, but she still asked. Even through the losses she did the best she could. It wasn't until after we chose to end IVF and learn how to accept the childfree life did she really struggle to get it. And ultimately, she struggled to really get me.

Throughout IVF, people will say the most insensitive and sometime downright rude things; however, most of them can be brushed off as simple ignorance. They just don't understand. The most hurtful words ever spoken to me were from this loved one and caught me so off-guard because they were so unexpected. In a small argument, Marie interrupted me and said the words she will never get to take back. The words that will be seared into my soul for a very long time.

"I am so tired of that fucking excuse! So what, you guys can't have kids, you CHOSE not to have kids! How long are we going to hear about it?"

An excuse?

A choice?

But, it IS my truth.

How long?

Unfortunately, my entire life as losing this dream is a lifelong loss.

I was so shocked by her words that I quickly ended the conversation and didn't even address it at that point. I was in complete disbelief that

---

3   Name has been changed for privacy.

someone, who I thought loved me unconditionally, would think, let alone say those words. Never in my life have I felt so hurt, so invalidated and disappointed.

She does not get it. And, she may never get it.

What the hell do I do with that?

For years, I have helped clients with accepting the limitations of their loved ones. That sometimes our loved ones, especially our families, just don't have what we need. Sometimes, they are incapable. It doesn't mean that we don't deserve it or that it isn't unfair. But the fact is that perhaps they are an empty well and the only way we will feel better is if we stop going to the empty well looking for water.

For probably a million reasons, Marie is not able to get what I have been through or what I will continue to go through, for the rest of my life. I found that her judgment and dismissal of my losses made me doubt myself, at first

Do I use this journey and what I have survived as an excuse to stay angry or bitter?

Do I just need to get over this?

I even took it as far as allowing her doubt to invalidate me and my story. What if the world thinks I didn't want kids bad enough because I stopped IVF treatments and know that adoption isn't for us?

This is when I knew I had to start taking my own advice, quite possibly the hardest thing for anyone to do, therapist or not. To practice what we preach. I had to start the work of accepting the limitations of Marie, and of others, who just don't have the capacity to get it or to get me. She is one of my incapables.

Throughout my life, I have always seen what trauma and hardship can do to our relationships. It can strengthen them or damage them, and sometimes it can even end them. Going through my back surgeries at ages fourteen and seventeen, I saw this with friends and family, both my own and of my parents. However, I didn't have the education, life experience or soul I do today. Surviving IVF, saying no to adoption and doing the work on accepting a childfree life, I have learned that traumas and hardships never stop affecting our relationships, for better and worse. Except now, I have the words for them.

I have been very lucky and blessed with the people who have stood by me throughout my life, at times pushing me from behind, walking alongside me or even pulling me forward. I have had people come in and out of my life time and again. I have lost some relationships throughout the hardships I have faced. But only after IVF and working on this childfree life, have I been able to determine my categories, or really, all categories of relationships.

• • • • •

My Fellow Warriors

My fellow warriors are those who have been through some version of infertility or pregnancy loss themselves, even if their journey has looked completely different (typically their outcome) than mine. My fellow warriors are also the people who have not walked in my shoes, but still have the understanding, they know loss of some kind. They choose to live their lives authentically and alongside with me.

My fellow warriors genuinely get it.

With them I am truly known.

• • • • •

My True Friends (Really Family)

My true friends are those who may have never had to think about infertility, never really been exposed to it and therefore struggle to empathize with my journey, but they still try. My true friends ask the questions, sometimes not in the best way, but they still ask.

My true friends walk along beside me.

With them I am truly seen.

• • • • •

My Limited Supporters

My limited supporters are those who will never ask about my journey and become extremely uncomfortable whenever it's brought up but they get every other aspect of my story, of me.

My limited supporters do the best with what they have.

With them I am truly loved.

• • • • •

My Incapables

My incapables are those who openly criticize, question and deny what we have been through. My incapables may have tried talking and asking about it, but have never quite had the capacity to understand any of it. Not only do they deny my journey, but often times somehow shut down that part of who I am.

My incapables will probably never get it.

With them I am incomplete.

• • • • •

These categories not only apply to my IVF journey, but rather, I think, they are what happens to all of us as we grow, evolve and love. Relationships change, relationships end, relationships reemerge, relationships evolve.

I use the term re-categorize with my clients a lot, referring to the ever-changing relationships in our lives as we age. I believe people are meant to come in and out of our lives as we all change. Sometimes these changes warrant a re-categorization. Some people you thought would always be there might leave your life for a few years and then reemerge, or they may be gone forever, never meant to be the lifelong friend you had hoped.

Hand in hand with re-categorization is accepting limitations. We all must accept the limitations of our loved ones. Sometimes, they just don't have what we need. Accepting their limitations improves our well-being, as we only have control over ourselves. We cannot *make* someone understand us. Accepting our loved ones' limitations means we realize they just don't have it to give. We must stop going to the empty well.

Being completely understood by others has nothing to do with who we are or our stories. We must honor ourselves, no matter what our loved ones' capabilities of understanding us are. *We all must do the work to validate ourselves; seeing, knowing and loving ourselves.*

Life is difficult and people are complicated, which means relationships take work and are forever changing.

Myself, I must accept that there are some people in my life who will *never* understand my journey of infertility or the lifelong losses in my childfree life. Even though this can feel like a complete denial of who I am and may change our relationship, I must continue to speak my truth and live my story authentically for the world to see, because this is simply who I am.

I must be my truth, not to fulfill the need to feel understood or to make someone get it, but rather to live my authentic truth and light.

To be true to myself.

For that light will reveal my fellow warriors and true friends.

The biggest lesson of my IVF and childfree journey?

Connection is what it is all about it. My relationships have been a huge part of my survival and continued thriving. Relationships are a major focus in positive psychology and research continues to demonstrate how relationships heal us all, making us better and happier people. My continued lesson is that this healing occurs not in spite of, but because of all my relationships: the fellow warriors, true friends, limited supporters and even the incapables. Relationships change and grow, because we change and grow.

The relationships I have with my limited supporters, and even the incapables, may not be my most poignant, meaningful or deep right now. But that doesn't mean they will remain that way forever. It may just mean that I need to limit how vulnerable I am with them, how much I let them into my life, and how much effort I put in, as they choose to simply not get it. They choose to not see me or know me, and therefore do not love me unconditionally. As Brené Brown, writes and speaks, "if you aren't 'daring greatly' in my arena, I'm not interested in your feedback". Brown often times quotes this excerpt from the Theodore Roosevelt speech "Citizenship in a Republic"

It is not the critic who counts;
not the man who points out how the strong man stumbles
or where the doer of deeds could have done better.

The credit belongs to the man who is actually in the arena,
whose face is marred by dust and sweat and blood,
who strives valiantly, who errs and comes up short again and again,
because there is no effort without error or shortcoming,
but who knows the great enthusiasms,
the great devotions,

who spends himself for a worthy cause;
who, at the best, knows, in the end, the triumph of high achievement,
and who, at the worst, if he fails, at least he fails while daring greatly…

I think the tough question, is what to do with our limited supporters and our incapables. We cannot make any of them understand us. We can only ask for what we want and need from them. We also cannot change our loved ones. We can only change the relationship in so much as changing ourselves. Therefore, there may be times that our relationships with the limited supporters and the incapables need to be set aside, because they do not honor us. They do not see us. They are unable to know us.

Things change, and people change. I've changed. This limited love and understanding may not be forever. The only thing I can do is to continue to live my authentic truth, asking for what I want and need from my loved ones, and accepting their limitations. Because one day, the incapable just might finally see my bravery in battle and decide to join me in the arena, but only if I never stop believing in my own "daring greatly" and ever upward.

Because our light, our path, our ever upward is in owning our story no matter the understanding we receive back.

Because only then will my relationships flourish instead of die, even in times of trauma and hardship.

Because only then, am I honoring myself and my story, therefore demanding the same from my loved ones.

Because only then, when I am happy and whole myself, am I able to nourish all of my relationships. My marriage included.

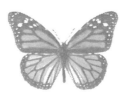

Chapter 6

Reigniting the Spark

O ne day, I hope there will be research published on the effect of infertility and IVF on marriages and relationships. Unfortunately, I suspect that the numbers could reflect major damage.

A typical scenario involves a couple trying for year(s) to have children. When that doesn't work, they continue trying for years with assisted fertility treatments; spending thousands and thousands of dollars, scheduling intercourse or fertilization and making sex the least romantic thing ever, dealing with terrible side effects and painful procedures that put more and more stress on the relationship. How could these traumas not have long-term effects on the relationship, despite the desired outcome of children?

IVF is difficult, much like any other major health crisis or dream crusher we survive in our lives. The only difference is that IVF involves both of us. Sure maybe the "cause" of infertility is the man's low sperm count, or perhaps the woman struggles with endometriosis, but no matter the cause, together they have trouble conceiving their lifelong wish of children. It was my doing that we couldn't conceive children naturally; my back surgeries and maybe even my fears, but Chad has always reassured me that he knew going in that we would figure it out. Never throughout our entire process did he ever outwardly blame me or make me feel at fault for our lack of a family. We were a team.

We are a team with a great balance, as I have written; me feeling everything and him being extremely balanced and even keeled, but we make it work together. Moving forward with our impossible decision of accepting a childfree life meant we also had to move through the grief process. Elizabeth Kubler-Ross wrote long ago about the stages of grief: denial, anger, bargaining, depression/feeling and, finally, acceptance. Helping many clients work their way through life after a major loss I have learned that these stages are never the same for anyone and they look can very different for each of us. They also don't necessarily happen in order and tend to work more on a spiral, sometimes even needing to repeat themselves time and time again.

Our grief was no different. I think some of it is personality difference and some of it simply gender difference. I feel a lot, I talk a lot and I express A LOT. Chad does not. Whether or not it is because he is a man or because that's just who he is doesn't matter. However, I have also concluded that a big part of it is also the circumstances of our IVF journey, losing our babies and accepting our childfree life. I felt all of it, all of the time and always very openly. I think this open expression shut down Chad's emotions at times, leaving him with the sense of needing to pull his shit together in order to remain strong for me and pick up my pieces.

Only after much conversation and feeling through all of this together, have we found our stride. We have been able to hear each other's voices, thoughts and feelings about all of it. The biggest piece about moving forward together was learning to redefine ourselves both as a non-father and non-mother but also as a couple and family. We started this part of our journey on a trip to Lake Tahoe.

We purposefully chose the end of July for our trip to get as close as possible to what would have been the first birthday of the two embryos from the first transfer. I can't say for certain why we chose Lake Tahoe, but there was just something that drew us there; we had always heard how beautiful it was. We spent five days hiking through some of the most magnificent mountains I have ever laid eyes on, sitting on the shorelines of beautiful crystal clear lakes, eating scrumptious food and drinking delectable wine in the sunshine while reconnecting. Really redefining. We found us again. Me, letting go of the anger and sadness, and Chad often pushing, sometimes pulling, but nevertheless walking along beside me the entire way. We had just made it through our own version of hell. We spent much of the trip pushing me through the strangling thin air to the top of that mountain while I bitched, complained, and probably yelled some, all the while Chad encouraged me and maintained course, it was the perfect metaphor for our early marriage. We pushed through to see the awe-inspiring crystal blue color of the lake that we were the only people on. We sat and reflected, separately and together.

I walked back into myself on that trip, which meant that I walked back into us.

We ended 2012 looking forward to our bright but tough rebuilding of 2013. For Christmas, I had absolutely no idea what to get Chad. He is one of the most difficult people to shop for; I will also completely admit that I am not the best gift giver, depending on the recipient. I would never buy him clothes because he is very meticulous with how

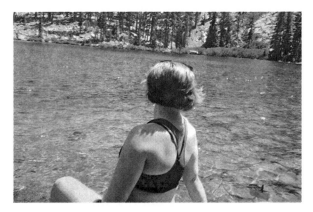

Redefining in Lake Tahoe.

things fit, although, thank God he is willing to take my input. He waved goodbye to those pleated pants as soon as we met! I would also never buy him electronics or tools, as he enjoys researching them a ton and I wouldn't want to take that away from him. I would also rather gifts be a surprise than someone telling me exactly what to get. A few searches on Pinterest and some reading of blogs later I found a blog post where a woman had pre-purchased and planned a year of dates for her and her husband. Brilliant! So that is what I set forth to do.

What better way to find ourselves again, bring us back to us, have fun and spend quality time together than to make sure we have a planned activity for every month of the coming year. I compiled my ideas, made a Word document all pretty with pictures and printed them out. I let him see the entire year planned out when he opened the gift and then we took each month and put it in a sealed envelope. On the first day of every month in 2013, we would open our envelope to see what that month's date was.

January – At Home Wine Tasting
I was a little anxious about our first date, I knew it would be fun because wine was involved, but I really wanted this idea to work for us, the first

step in a year of dates to help bring us back to us. I had so much fun preparing this date at home, I made some grading sheets and bought some dark salted caramel chocolates, cheese and crackers, grapes and ten bottles of wine under thirteen dollars each. I marked each bottle with its purchase price, and then hid it in a paper bag for a blind taste test. I included what we then thought was our favorite wine. I even managed to surprise Chad with my creativity.

For each tasting, we toasted to something meaningful or lighthearted before we took a sip, or two or three, of the wine. On our grading sheet, we each rated the wine on a scale of one to ten, with ten being the best wine we'd ever tasted. Then we each had to come up with one or two words to describe the wine. Chad and I laughed hysterically as we described the wines as ghostly, watery, young, light, and smooth. Our lists did not include many adjectives you'd hear from your favorite sommelier, but they were ours nonetheless. At the end of our very official tasting we were shocked to discover that what we thought was our favorite wine we found to be quite disgusting indeed, going so far as to describe it as soapy water. On the bright side, we found a new favorite that was a $9.99 bottle called Apothic Red. We laughed, we drank, we ate and we started the year off in our

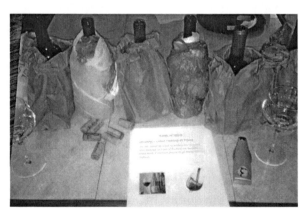

At home wine tasting.

way. Looking back, this laughter was the best way to start our year of healing dates, we had so much fun that we decided to make the at home wine tasting an annual tradition.

February – Game Night at Home
The anticipation leading up to our second date of 2013 started building a few days before. With the smell of competition in the air, we put on our most comfortable workout clothes and spent the evening competing against each other in Wii games. I was sure that a lifetime of dancing combined with my Wii *Just Dance* skills would really pull out the win for me. The loser of this month's date had to empty the dishwasher for two weeks. We played several Wii sports and then moved on to *Wii Sports Resort*, which always ends up in hilarity. We laughed with and at each other, at how silly we looked, and at the dogs, especially Gertie and Gracie who love to jump and pounce around with each other, playing alongside us.

Chad's decathlete athleticism could not be contained for long and he definitely beat me in the Wii sports games, but if it had been only *Just Dance*, no doubt he would have been emptying the dishwasher! This month's date was a great reminder that games should not be solely reserved for those times we have company. Instead of watching television, on separate couches, we could engage with each other through friendly competition. Even though I had to empty the dishwasher for two weeks, I knew we had both won on so many levels.

March – Fancy Date Night – The Book of Mormon
Since we'd completed two at home dates, we figured it was time for a fancy date night. We scoured StubHub for reasonably priced tickets to the fabulous Fox Theater here in Saint Louis. It is definitely one of the fanciest (read *expensive*) dates we've had, but was an amazing

night out. We both worked that day, so we dressed up separately and met for a nice dinner at a new restaurant before heading to the show. At the theater, we saw *The Book of Mormon*. As the lights dimmed and the curtain went up, I felt like I was on a first date with Chad. If you don't know anything about the show, it's from the creators of Comedy Central's *South Park,* which is very politically incorrect. The cast's voices were simply amazing and the show was hysterical. Admittedly, I cringed a few times when the open minded, all accepting, empathic therapist part of my brain was shocked but I couldn't deny the humor and talent in the entire show. Chad of course, loved it! We drove home together, and again I was reminded of when we first started dating. I felt like we had really connected that night and felt a true spark.

April – Traditional Date Night – Dinner and a Movie
We upgraded our traditional date night of dinner and a movie and splurged for the dine-in theater. We required nothing fancy for dinner this month, and we didn't know what the food would be like at the dine-in theater, plus I cannot pass up movie theater popcorn with butter, one of my rare splurges, so we stopped by Buffalo Wild Wings. I was literally like an excited kid once we walked into the theater; our own plush leather reclining seats with our own pull around tables, cup holders and a full bar. Definitely a luxurious way to see a movie, and the only way I will see one now! To top it off we saw one of my favorite types of movies: a sports movie with a human-interest storyline, *42*. It was amazing! For someone who has never been sport inclined, we often joke that flying balls will usually end up hitting me in the face or head, I love a good sports movie. At one point in the evening, I looked over at Chad and saw the adoration in his eyes that he reserves for when I get really excited about something. I remembered why we fell in love in the first place. Underneath the strong team we have built ourselves into,

is the pure unadulterated adoration we have for who the other person genuinely is. It was a great night, and a good reminder that your dates don't necessarily have to take a ton of planning or money to be enjoyed or foster a deeper connection.

May – Hiking and a Picnic

We spent the day walking the trails at our favorite spot, Castlewood Park. The views are beautiful and the trails aren't too difficult, but far from boring. I was really looking forward to a picnic lunch, but it had rained the day before and the park was super wet and muddy, so we opted to grab brunch out. Hiking is always a great way for us to connect and something we've done often throughout our courtship and our marriage. I love our hikes together, pausing every so often to bask in the beauty of nature. Chad lets me stop to take pictures and we often attempt to take selfies, which never turn out due to our massive height difference. Our hikes usually include a friendly competition of light running and bets on when I will fall on my ass, just our running joke of how clumsy I am. We talked, laughed and walked/ran/hiked in silence. Sometimes the best quality time isn't filled with words but the strongest sense of connection can be found in stillness.

And this is where we let life get in the way… Like many couples busy with work, or even those who get too busy with their children, we fell off the wagon for a bit. We were in the middle of remodeling Mason House and we spent many evenings and weekends working on the property. Mason House and an unexpected injury got in the way of our scheduled date, so we postponed June and moved onto July. The work on Mason House, as grueling, gross, hot, bloody and obviously accident prone as it was, was something we did together every day and night that summer. A longed after goal and hard work made for some great dates night, some with the epic emotionality of a soap opera.

July – Casino Night

There are simply no sufficient words to describe how much I loathe gambling. But, Chad loves to play a few hands of blackjack, especially with me because he basically gets to play two hands at once. I cannot stand that smoking is still allowed in casinos. As someone who took Wellbutrin for years to manage my depression, I think I've developed a lifelong aversion to the smell of smoke. Casinos also tend to be full of people who are very alone or addicted, which the therapist in me has way too much empathy and motivation to help. Finally, I just don't get why I would want to give someone else the money I worked so hard to make! Nevertheless, I knew the casino had a great restaurant, so it was bound to be a good date night. We ate a delicious meal and each gambled twenty-five dollars at the blackjack tables. I'm always the more conservative one and want to walk away sooner than Chad, which is surprising for us, as he is definitely the smarter and more conservative spender. He coached me the entire time, because I just don't give enough shits to learn the game. Blackjack has always been something where we work great as a team. I know how much he loves the game but doesn't get to play it often; he knows I literally have a mental block to learning it. And so we make a great team. He is able to coach me through. It is in times like these that I am reminded, and saddened that he will never get to teach our child something new. Within that silly moment in a smoky casino, I see the time, attention and love in his teaching. We didn't win big, but we didn't lose either; we came home with twenty dollars in each of our wallets and love in our hearts.

August – Slumber Party at Home

It worked out perfectly that we got to spend this date in our new home with the fireplace roaring. We each had plenty of advance notice to pick a movie that the other hadn't seen before. I knew exactly what movie I would make him watch: a classic, at least to my sister and me, *Drop*

Dead Fred. Chad should have had an easier time picking a movie, as I have never seen some of the major classics. People are always shocked by the fact that I have never seen *Goonies*, or any of the *Star Wars*, *Back to the Future* or *Indiana Jones* movies. I think it must have been growing up with only a sister; we were just never into those kinds of movies. After searching all over for whatever one was free or the cheapest, Chad finally decided on the first *Back to the Future*. We ate take out and way too much movie candy and enjoyed our movies by firelight. I'm not sure Chad loved *Drop Dead Fred* as much as I do, other than thinking it was hysterical that I still knew all the words. I, however, absolutely adored *Back to the Future* and couldn't wait to watch the sequels. August's movie date was our first really relaxing night in our new house, really solidifying our family's home in our new house.

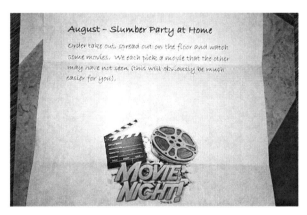

Movie night.

June – Driving Range

It was really September at this point, but we set out for our June date. I had suffered a chip fracture on my index finger working on the yard of our new house and couldn't golf back in June, but by September, I was good to go. I've never really hit golf balls before, except for the occasional mini-golf, which again I will reiterate; I'm just terrible with balls. Chad enjoys golfing but only manages to get to the course twice a year if he's lucky. It was a crisp, clear fall day so we went to the driving range and hit a couple buckets of balls. Chad showed me how to hold the club, taught me how to hit and tried to educate me on the different club types. Before IVF, we would have struggled for him to teach me something new. It was almost as if we both brought in too much bravado. However, one major blessing of IVF is how much better we work as a team, even when it means that one of us has to teach the other something new. I wouldn't say I am going pro any time soon, but at least we had an amazing afternoon together.

September – Cardinals Baseball Game
Once again, we let life distract us. We didn't open our September envelope until the end of October, which meant that it was post-season baseball. In 2013 that meant the World Series for the AMAZING St. Louis Cardinals. Needless to say, we couldn't quite score World Series tickets within our budget so we prepped to watch the game at home. We dressed in our Cardinal's red, ordered hot wings to go and cheered on the Redbirds with all our might. For dessert, instead of cotton candy at the ballpark, we settled for fireplace s'mores at home. It was a stressful game, but fun and way cheaper than eight-dollar ballpark beers.

October – Murder Mystery Dinner
I loathe Halloween and have as long as I can remember. However, tell me a good ghost story and you have my attention! One of our favorite Sunday brunch places in Saint Louis is the Lemp Mansion. Lemp Mansion is the historical site of the Lemp family brewery and is chock full of history, including several reported suicides which of course means reported paranormal activity. Year-round they host murder mystery dinners where the costumes are corny and the acting so-so, but the food delicious and the bar open. Plus, it is held within the hauntingly

(literally) beautiful walls of the mansion. In the spirit of Halloween, we got tickets to their murder mystery dinner for our October date. We met for happy hour after work before heading down into the city, and again it felt the old days when we were dating, before the pressure of IVF. We were having such a great conversation that we ended up having one glass of wine too many and were almost late for the murder mystery dinner. We arrived right before dinner, which meant we got small parts. However, Chad's character name made up for it. That and the fact he had to wear his name tag all night ...Tu Long Dong.

November – Shopping Date
Believe it or not, I am also not a huge fan of shopping and never have been. Now give me the credit card and my favorite websites and I can online shop for hours! But Chad hardly ever shops for himself, so I knew planning a shopping date would allow us to spend a few hours together updating his wardrobe, which he desperately needed because he hates shopping just as much as I do. We checked out one of our new fancy outlet malls here in Saint Louis and updated much of his closet. I did not get one thing for myself, except of course my forbidden mall hot pretzel smothered in salt. Worth the cheat on my meal plan every time! As I savored my pretzel, I realized that before IVF this date wouldn't have been nearly as successful or fun for us. I was grateful for everything we have been through because we are so much more connected and in tune with each other now.

December – Winter Wonderland
The Winter Wonderland Light display at Tillis Park is famous in Saint Louis every holiday season. In my eleven years in Saint Louis, I had never once gone through the display. This year, we used our year of dates to check it out, finally. I splurged for our own private horse drawn carriage to take us through the park, although we had some unexpected guests.

Earlier that week, we found out that one of our favorite restaurants was closing down at the end of the week, due to retirement. We often frequented this beloved restaurant with our friends Clint and Janine, and their three boys. So for our last favorite garlic laced meal in Saint Louis we invited Clint and Janine on our December date. Our horse drawn carriage tickets were for four people anyways. We went to dinner, laughed our butts off, ate garlic to our hearts desire and then we all bundled up and headed to the park. It was actually nice to have another couple with us; we finally got some good pictures of us on our monthly date! Clint and Janine are our family. They have been amazing support to us throughout our journey and we love their boys so much. It was fitting that we ended our year of dates with them tagging along.

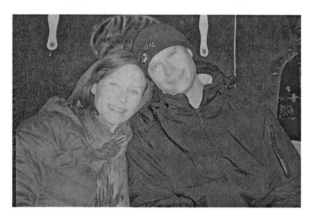

Winter Wonderland.

The year of dates helped Chad and I to remember to make our relationship a priority. It also helped us to figure out what our family is, for us. Some people may not consider a childfree couple as a family, or even our dogs as our children. However, this is our family. We love each other just as much as the childfull family does. We have traditions just like the childfull family does. And we matter just as much as the childfull family does.

Throughout the year, I continued my vulnerability, connection and using social media in a positive way and posted our monthly dates. I found that so many people loved the ideas and contributed great ideas for the future. I also had several people ask if they could steal the idea, to which I obviously said of course, I did the very same myself. I hope that we were able to show our friends and families, even the busy ones with several kids that making time for each other, even if it's just once a month, is important. We had fun. We connected and dated again, something that every long-term couple needs to remember to put effort into.

Marriages and partnerships, just like relationships, will either evolve and flourish or wither and die in times of trauma and hardship. Each partner must do his or her own work on healing in addition to working together. We both must be happy, healthy and whole to be a happy and healthy couple. Throughout our journey of IVF and the acceptance of our childfree life, I am coming to believe that this evolvement and flourishing is more of a choice than some would like to believe. I think Chad and I could have very easily let our losses, heartbreaks and financial difficulties from IVF come between us, but we have chosen to come together and do the work to make it all help us grow us into a stronger couple. Communication and trust are huge in this process, but so is laughter. Our year of dates was a huge part of creating this strength. Our survival of IVF gave us the foundation to grow together. This foundation prepared us for the building of our dream, our family, our home, our Mason House.

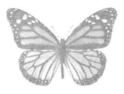

Chapter 7

Building Our Family Home

When we began our IVF journey, Chad and I bought a pink house in a family friendly suburb of Saint Louis because we wanted to be closer to our support system, we wanted to be closer to our friends with kids, and because the school districts were ranked highest in the Saint Louis area. We also totally thought the house was white until we got our first snow and realized, nope, it's pretty damn pink! We made this decision without the knowledge that IVF would not work for us, and ultimately that fancy school district was to be wasted on a childfree couple. Our now famous pink house helped us build stronger relationships with our friends since we were so close to them and their support helped us tremendously during our IVF journey and afterwards.

When our journey ended, without the intended, hoped for and prayed for result of children, we no longer needed the suburban environment. As a woman without children, I stuck out like a sore thumb; no soccer practices to attend and no minivan meant I just didn't fit in. We had dreamt of owning a house with a pool one day, and this dream only strengthened after our IVF journey ended and we decided to learn how to accept a childfree life. I knew in my heart that having a pool would help us stay connected with our friends and all of their children. We could be the fun house where everyone came all summer long. We could be part of their growing up. However, I will also admit I wanted a pool because I didn't want to be forgotten about or left behind.

After much consideration, we knew it just wasn't a good decision to put a pool in at pink house. Pools aren't great investments, but it really wasn't a good investment in our neighborhood that already had a subdivision pool and our backyard just wasn't quite private enough. So, we did some random searches. What can't you add? You can't add land. We searched for properties with land in the Saint Louis area. We looked in a more central location, not necessarily in family-ville USA. After we stumbled upon a property that looked intriguing, I drove by it and just had that feeling. I had to convince Chad to even look at the property; a midcentury home on an acre of land in the middle of Saint Louis. The kicker was that it would be a gut rehab since it hadn't been touched since the 1950's.

First, we had to sell pink house and we had to sell it at a certain price, especially after the financial hardship of IVF, to be even ready to forge forward with this dream. We met with a realtor who specialized in our subdivision and got our list of must-get-done's before placing the house on the market. When we asked her when we needed to go on the market, her response was last week. We worked our asses off and got pink house on the market in a week. Our open house was on a Sunday; a house down the street well above our price range went on the market on that Wednesday and immediately got six offers, not even making it to their open house. There were five families disappointed and Chad and I hoped that would work in our favor. We drove around town with the three dogs that Sunday during our open house and had two offers that night. Things were falling in place fast; the magic had begun.

We received two contracts the next day. We were moving and moving soon.

That day, we made an appointment to see that cute midcentury home on the acre of land. As we walked through the house we both could see the vision, but we kept looking over at the property next door, which was also on the market with the same realtor. She said she would be happy to show us that house... *however, there were some challenges.* It was an 'as is property' owned and currently lived in by a woman who struggles with hoarding. The house had the exact same layout except for a few additions; an extra bathroom and a walkout basement to a condemned pool. The layout of the land also provided a lot more usable space. I will never forget Chad's face when he looked at me and said, "Turn off the therapist part of your head; we are going to look at this house. It's $80,000 cheaper and may need the same amount of work this one does." Across the front yards, we walked, and into our cluttered future, we stumbled.

Between Chad and I, we had bought and sold five houses at this point in our relationship. We were masters at it really. But, never have I been able to walk into a space and see my vision or our family home. The traumas of IVF and the loss of three babies somehow changed everything about my filters. For the first time ever, I walked into a property and was able to see past what was there to what was meant to be there for us; our family home.

Joan[4], the owner of the home was there while we walked through with the realtor. She was tattered looking and very thin, but full of

---

4   Name has been changed for privacy.

kindness and love. The house was full, up to Chad's shoulders full, with only a walking path through the main living area. Full from floor to ceiling, two floors and about four thousand square feet full of fifty years of things. Things dirty with dust, but nothing too gross at first sight. The layout of the house was perfect and the property even better. Looking around at the foundation and the bones of the house it appeared to be in great shape. Both houses would need to be completely gut rehabbed, so we would spend a comparable amount of money on the finished product no matter which house we chose. Why not spend a significantly less amount on the purchase price? But, we knew we needed to get a contractor to tell us this could be done for our budget, that it was not too crazy and actually doable.

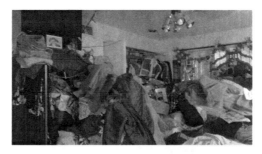

The full master bedroom.

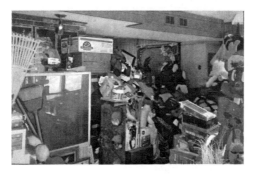

The full great room.

Looking back on that time, I do not have the words for the magic I felt. There was never a time that both Chad and I lost sight of our vision for the house. There was just something about it, our future, our dream, our family home within this house that sat on Mason road. Therein we found our Mason House and felt home deep in our hearts and souls. Throughout the next five months, we never lost this feeling, despite some of the worst luck and many frustrations during the purchase and construction processes. We kept our vision the entire time. We had hope and love, and with it we built Mason House.

We started with one contractor who told us our dream was actually feasible. I will never forget when we walked through the still floor-to-ceiling-full-of-things-house with him. Every so often, he would stop and attempt to pull things out to get a better look at the structure of the house. Down in the basement or as we will forever refer to it, the bowling alley, because it is so long and would make a perfect two lane bowling alley, he inspected the foundation. "No cracks, beautiful headers," he stated, "they just don't build homes like this anymore." In that one statement, he had just given us the green light we needed.

During this time, we were also moving out of pink house. That sale had everything go wrong and was the most difficult sale we have ever had, yet we both knew it was meant to be. We trusted, we struggled and we fought for our dream. We moved out of pink house into an eight hundred square foot short-term lease apartment that was just five minutes away from Mason House. Most everything we owned went into storage while the three dogs and us played college again and moved back to apartment living.

The contract negotiations on the house were not easy, but we got through it. During this waiting period, we had three house contractors and three pool contractors meet with us at Mason House one Saturday as Joan went out looking for a new condo. Our realtor, Jim, had to sit with us that day within the chaos and filth of Mason House. We were there for seven hours, most of it without heat, in March. Each contractor walked through the property asking what we would like to do to the house, the timeline, etc. The pool contractors all inspected the condemned pool to ask what we envisioned for our own. The pool was an old concrete pool that hadn't been cared for in probably thirty years. It literally had a forest growing out of it. Most people would walk out into the yard and ask where the pool was while they were looking right at it. Unless the pool was specifically pointed out to people, it was easily missed in the uncared forest of our acre yard.

Sometime during the contractor day at the house, we also had the sewer inspection, in which we learned she had been living without water for a "few years." The water backed up when we turned it back on, but the sewer inspection, which could have been the deal breaker, was not catastrophic. Spending seven hours in, hopefully, our future forever home we only continued to get more excited with our vision, despite with how much work and effort this project was going to take. The history of the house was beginning to unravel and the treasures inside only intrigued us more. We also began to forge a strange relationship with Joan.

From what we guessed, the house next door went on the market and Joan, knowing she had not paid her taxes in three years and her house would be going on auction in August, decided to use the same realtor to put hers on the market too. She had inherited the home from her mother who passed in 2006. Joan was always very kind to us. She always called us babe, and if the only thing I needed to do to get into to heaven was to be God blessed by Joan, I would have a first class ticket waiting for me. Ultimately, the therapist in me knew this process was impossible for her. She was losing her childhood home and quite possibly everything in it. Her realtor attempted to help her have several sales to sell some of her belongings, as there was no money left and there was no way she would be able to take everything in the house with her to her new condo. The sales never went well, and it was then that her realtor recommended adding a clause to our contract in hopes of motivating her to clear out the property. A $5,000 penalty was added stating that Joan would have to pay the penalty at closing if she didn't have the property cleaned out. This also meant that whatever was left in the home upon closing would be ours. We all hoped this would provide her with motivation to get the house emptied. Unfortunately, I knew all too well she was just too sick for this. And I couldn't help but be the therapist I am and fight for her.

We let Joan's realtor know we would be interested in purchasing some of her things to keep in the house and that my parents, avid flea market goers and antique hobbyists, would also like to purchase a few pieces. The first time we had set to meet with her, she changed her mind at the last minute. The second time, we came over and walked through the house and I saw for the first time just how sick she truly was. Everything we asked about had a story. She never could name a price of what she would part with the item for. The Elvis whiskey decanter my dad asked her about was not for sale because her deceased brother looked like Elvis. Finally, we came across the item that shut it down for me; my mom asked her about a porcelain tower of elephants from the Saint Louis Zoo. My niece loves elephants, as my mom informed Joan and asked her how much she would like for the figurine. My mom took the ceramic drama mask that was hanging on the tower of elephants off and picked up the tower to ask Joan how much she would like for it. Joan responded that they loved the Saint Louis Zoo growing up and besides where would she hang *her*, meaning the mask, if she sold us that? It was in that moment that I knew she would never get the house emptied, even though it had been on the market for several months. It was also in that moment that I couldn't not fight for her.

That night I emailed our unique and awkward story, with pictures, to two television hoarder shows. I was having difficulty finding resources in our area and hoped that the shows could at least provide me with some resources. Less than ten hours later, one called me back. I was beyond impressed with the treatment and the support Joan would get if she allowed the show to come tape her. Not only would they help her empty at least one room for the taping of the show, but they would provide her with a therapist and an organizer for a full six weeks after taping to help her finish the house. Additionally, she would receive a significant stipend to help her with aftercare. The naïve, but hopeful side of me wondered how anyone could turn down this much help. But, the realistic therapist in me knows that we all prefer our known dysfunction over the difficult work of change. But I tried anyways. Admittedly, I tried at least one time too many. All communication was through the realtor, unfortunately, but that was just the circumstances of our situation. I begged her to make Joan just call the show back and give permission to hear about the opportunity of help waiting for her. My last desperate plea to the realtor was simply that I was scared to death that come the day of closing, I would have to have Joan physically removed and arrested from the property and that I knew this would be more traumatic for her than it already was going to be. I also knew that she had several guns in the home and the paranoid part of me was scared of her desperation. The realtor, and Joan, assured me that her mom was the hoarder, not her, and that she didn't need any help. Chad looked at me that night and said, "You have to stop; she isn't going to accept the help." I knew he was right, but I knew I wouldn't be honoring myself if I hadn't tried that last time.

We moved forward with the closing on Mason House, knowing that most likely we would also be inheriting all of the belongings with it. Never in our wildest dreams did we imagine that this wouldn't be the most stressful part of rehabbing a home formerly owned by a hoarder. Three days before closing, our bank started getting nervous about our terrible appraisal. The appraisal came in so low that we had to readjust the purchase price. We think one of two things happened. Either the appraiser just could not see past all the crap in the home to see the potential that it held once emptied and remodeled or he had an investor on the side that wanted to tear down the house and was hoping our deal would fall through. So three days before closing our bank told us they would only do the loan with 5% more down. After IVF, we simply did not have that kind of money sitting in the bank. So, I made the phone call that I had dreaded my entire life. Barely able to catch my breath to speak, I called my parents asking for a loan. I was filled with shame and fear; shame that I needed to ask for financial help, and fear that we were going to lose this dream. Both of our parents helped with Mason House. Again, a testament to the power of what this house really meant to all of us. Needless to say, the bank was surprised that we were able to pull it off. We closed on Mason House just a couple of days after the original closing date.

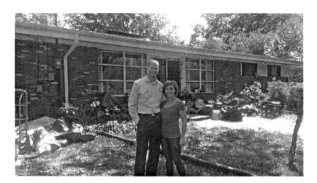

Closing day!

Joan signed her papers and we signed ours, then off we headed to the house to see what kind of progress she made emptying the property. She was still "packing" up some things that evening. We allowed her to stay for one hour after the funds transferred. Seeing the sad desperation in her realization that this was over for her, we agreed to let Joan come back that next day for one hour after we got off work, as we were going to be at the house getting at least one of the bathrooms cleaned out. We had friends and family descending over a three-day weekend to help us empty the house so we wanted to make sure we had a clean, working bathroom ready for them. We also wanted Joan to have her first night in her new condo, just in case she remembered or needed anything else. We felt that we had to do this, as there was clearly no rhyme or reason in what she packed. From what we could tell, she literally only took what she could see.

That next day we met my in laws at the house after work to empty out and clean at least one of the bathrooms. Joan came back with a helper that her realtor had hired to help her. We gave her one hour to continue "packing." As we worked, separately for the most part, we could overhear Joan and her helper some. As we emptied the bathrooms, we found endless boxes of unopened Kleenex, boxes of unused and expired hand sanitizer and diabetes supplies. Both showers and all the cabinets were full. It was shocking and sad but insanely funny at the same time. We filled a 1/8 of a 30-yard dumpster with just two small bathrooms. Everything we set out to donate to Goodwill, Joan would eventually remember she needed it and pack it away for her new condo.

As her hour began to end, you could feel her desperation fill the stale air of the house and the tension rise. At one point, we heard her helper yell out, "You owe me $20 dollars!"

"What? No, I don't!" she replied.

"Remember, no cursing here! These people are nice enough to let you back into THEIR home to go through THEIR stuff and take it. Be respectful, no cussing!" he yelled back.

She mumbled something back to him and it was quiet for the next ten minutes or so.

At the end of her hour, her helper had her come and thank Chad and I in person. With tears in her eyes she thanked us for letting her come back. She reminded us to watch our dogs on the busy street and of course blessed us and called us babe, like she had for the last several weeks. She then mumbled something to the effect that if we ever saw her again she would be wearing the exact same thing because she didn't get to pack any clothes. Her helper interrupted her and said, "No, you had months to do that, just thank them."

All the while, we were thinking, you've had your house on the market for months; you've had plenty of time to pack. That, and NO we will never see you again! Even though, we both knew this was never your traditional house purchasing situation, and that most likely we would see Joan several more times.

They left the house, in separate vehicles to meet back at her new condo. Less than five minutes later, Joan was back in the house claiming she had lost her car keys.

She lost her car keys in a hoarder's home! We helped her retrace her steps; trying to keep her on track and not letting her pack anything else. She held a black trash bag and kept trying to sneak things into it. She spotted an important black file cabinet and had to look in the drawers. It only contained more crap, but also her social security card. As she pulled the drawers out and dumped them into the black trash bag, Chad asked, "Joan, don't you want to put that somewhere safe?"

"This is safe."

We kept reminding her that her helper was waiting for her at her new place and was going to be very angry with her if we didn't find her keys and get her going soon. It took us at least twenty minutes to find them. All the while, reminding her that this isn't her house any more or that these things were now ours, and that she couldn't take anything else with her or we would have to call the cops. In fourteen years of working in mental health, I have never seen such desperation, sadness and illness that up close. And I wasn't even in my office or in an agency; I was in my new home. It was one of the most difficult hours of my fourteen year career.

We worked late into the night with the help of Chad's parents, Jim and Terry. We laughed, we cursed (well mostly me) and we smelled terrible. But, we got two of the bathrooms emptied and clean enough to use.

An eighth of a dumpster and only two of the smallest rooms were cleared out!

The next day the troops descended. My parents came down from Iowa with tons of supplies and food to get us through the weekend of emptying almost 4,000 square feet of a hoarder's paradise and our hell. We had friends and family come from near and far to help with the endeavor. Never have I ever felt more loved, believed in and grateful.

It was the hottest, smelliest and hardest work I'm sure most of us have ever experienced, and yet it was a ton of fun, full of laughter and utter disbelief.

We set up a system.

Under a couple of tents, we set up chairs, the yummy food my mom brought and coolers full of beer and water. Every hour or two, I would enforce a drink break. Everyone had to sit down, drink a whole bottle of water and rest.

We set up assembly lines outside the entrances to the home. Some people carried things out of the house. Some people stood in the assembly line just to go through everything. Whomever came across the item became the judge and had to determine if the item was donate, throw away, or a cool vintage item to be set aside for us to decide to keep or sell. It would take on average at least an hour for someone to acclimate to the system. At one point, I had to interrupt my friend Kelly after an hour of her just going through things muttering to herself, "holy shit, holy shit, holy shit!" over and over. "Kelly, I know this is crazy," I said, "but we have three days to empty out this entire house. Don't over think it; just go with your gut: trash, donate or keep."

We had tarps set up all across the back yard, each became a pile for trash, donate or keep. For the trash we would fill cans full of the non-salvageable contents of the house, load them onto a small trailer and then pull the trailer around to the front of the house to the dumpster.

We used Chad's car to pull the trailer, his Honda Pilot. The car he had bought because he was excited at how big it was. "It can hold two sheets of plywood, Babe!"

To which I replied, "It kind of looks like a mom car."

And here we were at our hoarder house that we bought because I would never be a mom, using the mom car to empty the house.

At this point, mostly Chad and Chad only, would empty the cans into the thirty-yard dumpsters, over and over and over again. Tall, athletic Chad never really got to enjoy the treasure hunting, as he was best utilized as manpower to unload the trailer.

There were definitely ground rules, especially because you just never knew what you would find. We were convinced that there just had to be treasures and you never know where people are inclined to hide money!

1. Every piece of clothing needed to be inspected and every pocket emptied.
2. Every envelope, file, and folder torn open and each side looked at.
3. Every picture frame torn apart.
4. Every drawer emptied, taken out and inspected underneath.
5. Every corner of every carpet pulled up to inspect.
6. Every purse and every crevice of that purse looked in.
7. Everything turned inside out, ripped open and inspected.

The house was filled with almost 4,000 square feet of very old electronics, furniture, clothing in every size, hundreds of never worn shoes and purses in every size, shape and color, and just things, some really crazy things.

We kept a lot of the furniture. We refinished some beautiful barrel chairs, we cleaned up an extended Saginaw table and I chalk painted some end tables and a couple of dressers. Most of the furniture had water damage from sitting in the basement for years, and some even had mold. Some were salvageable, some were not and some I had to paint, much to the irritation of my parents who have a strong love and appreciation for antiques. We found some pieces that we learned were worth some money, but we wanted to keep as much in the house as possible, hopefully combining the old with the new.

One such piece was a very low coffee table we found in the garage. Joan had set many of her things on it and used it to support a clothing rack at one point. It was severely water damaged, so we didn't even bother to look it up online, thinking it would never be worth anything. We had a corner table that seemed to be by the same designer. The corner end table was in pristine condition, and we had already planned to use it in the house. But, the low coffee table was the perfect step stool for Chad as he emptied the trashcans in to the huge dumpster. It sat outside for all three days of emptying on the house and then some. It wasn't until months later, when Chad and I were out shopping at a local mid-century antique store that we discovered who designed both pieces. The antique store had a buffet that was in beautiful condition and looked just like our corner table and the low coffee table. The designer was Paul Frankl and the buffet's list price was $5,500! We asked for advice on the restoring the corner table and if Frankl's pieces always sold for this much.

Then we tortured ourselves by attempting to find the low coffee table online, just to see what it may have been worth. Chad finally found it and we were shocked. In beautifully restored pristine condition, the table had sold for over $14,000. Where was our coffee table you ask?

Long gone, in a dumpster, like four dumpsters ago. It definitely stung. But, it is one of our best Mason House stories to date. We emptied everything in that house; we looked up everything that might've been worth anything. We never really found a major monetary treasure and all we had to do was just look down at the step stool we used the first weekend we emptied the house! I won't lie; it still stings some. When I told my best friend Lindsay about the potential value of the coffee table, she was shocked, "You mean to tell me, we looked in every pocket of every piece of clothing, every envelope, every file for even just a one dollar bill and we threw out a table worth thousands of dollars?!?!?"

"Yep."

The theme throughout the process of emptying Mason House was a high-pitched scream or squeal. As we all worked tirelessly in the heat, every so often we would hear the occasional squeal. The squeal could mean a few things.

1. Someone found something gross, like a dead mouse or live mice in which case the squealing was excessive but hilarious.
2. Someone found some cash or what he or she thought was a treasure.
   a. At the end of it, we found several hundred dollars that she left in the bottom of purses, still in the bank envelopes.
   b. We also were able to sell a few thousand dollars' worth of items to vintage stores in town or in small yard sales that we held.
3. Someone found something crazy or super weird.
   a. Blue crocheted nifty nipple warmers.
   b. A toothbrush with breasts on it.
   c. Odd books like *Sex After Death* or *Witch's Brew: Good Spells for Great Sex*.

    d. A bag of dildos.

    e. A small box of super old marijuana.

    f. A gun or bullets.

    g. More shoes that had never been worn.

    h. Or, when we finally dug our way to the mysterious tree in the middle of the basement. They had hollowed out a huge tree trunk to put around the beam in the basement. Then they actually stapled fake branches all along the ceiling.

4. Finally, I squealed with major delight as I was working on the last bathroom in the basement by myself on the last day with our family and friends helping. In that bathroom alone, I found an inflatable houseguest, 17 boxes (still shrink-wrapped) of a cheap golf gift set and no less than seven boxes of marbled mirror glass tiles. When I finally reached the shower at the back of the bathroom I stopped, looked up with my hand on the shower door and prayed loudly, "God, please let this shower be empty." I pulled the door open and squealed loudly, in delight… nothing! It was empty!

It was a true treasure hunt, a tough but funny hunt that we were all extremely blessed to experience together. The things we found will never be forgotten, even though most of it ended up in a landfill or at Goodwill. At one point, we were kicked out of a Goodwill store. The manager graciously thanked us and said how much he loved what we were bringing him, as most of it was brand new and just needed cleaning up, but they just didn't have any more space or manpower to continue taking our donations.

- Books, like old literature and poetry collections.
- Old cameras, video equipment and reels of film.

- Hundreds of bottles of liquor, most only about half full because the alcohol had evaporated so much in the last thirty years.
- Enough furniture for two houses.
- A pile of clothing that filled the entire living room up to the ceiling.
- Hundreds of pairs of unworn shoes all in size 9 (I'm a size 6.5!!!).
- An old, but still working, salon hair dryer chair.
- A swim cap with a blonde wig sewn into it.
- Trinkets. Millions of knick knacks and trinkets.
- China and hundreds of glasses.
- Dancing Elvis dolls that sang *Blue Christmas* – six of them.
- Plush *Playboy* bunny figurines holding martini glasses, all still in the box, all eight of them.
- Purses; purses with clocks built in, purses with a telephone built in, purses in every color and every size.
- Two old sewing machines.
- Probably at least a mile of random orange extension cords.
- Three disco balls, two of them unopened in the original packaging.
- Over 50 different decorations from *Pier 1* never taken out of the shopping bag, including at least 30 huge Christmas candles.
- Life size Christmas decorations.
- Hundreds of records and two record players, including a working Edison.
- Boxes upon boxes of costume jewelry.
- Shit. Not literal, thank God, just a bunch of crappy things that would never mean anything to anyone but to Joan and her mom in their unhealthy emotional entrapment in things.

It was sad. It was shocking. It has made for an amazing story. Our amazing story.

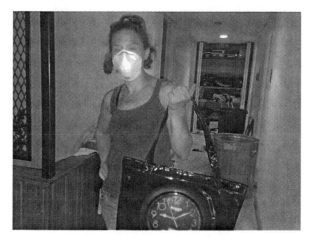

*Me and one of the hundreds of purses found
in the home, no money in this one.*

To thank our 13 friends and family who helped us those few days in the hard, dirty but amazingly fun work of emptying Mason House I bought them each a stepping stone kit. They could decorate them however they wished, we just wanted their names on it. When the pool and fire pit are complete, we will place the stepping-stones around them and those thirteen people will become a permanent part of Mason House. There are simply not sufficient words to thank them enough for their help, and to express how much it meant to us.

400 rubber gloves.

200 masks.

7 seventeen-foot trailer loads to Goodwill.

10 thirty-yard dumpsters…

…and Mason House was empty.

We held a weekend of sales to see if we could sell some of our found treasures and the most random people stopped by. One woman from the neighborhood came at least ten times in four days, and she always bought something. We will always remember her as the woman with the most unusual purchase. Throughout the emptying process we found a plethora of stuffed animals, some literally life sized. Each time we uncovered a critter, my dad took it to the front of the house and positioned it in a tree or in the front yard or even on the roof. When the house was empty there were several Care Bears in the trees, a lion on the roof and a life sized stuffed dog at the base of a tree. This neighbor woman, as I was helping her load her car with her third load at least turned to me and asked quietly, "Is the dog for sale?"

"But, it's been sitting outside for a few days. Even in the rain, I think." I replied.

"That's okay."

"Can I ask what you want it for?"

I will never ever forget the seriousness in her face as she replied, "Just to brush it and play with it."

"Oh! Of course, you can just have it."

To each their own.

It was also during the sale that we met a hysterical older couple from Peru. They bought us out of many things as they often send toys to children in other countries. They bought an amazing keyboard for their own granddaughter. They kept eyeing all the Japanese inspired furniture we had for sale, which was a lot. The husband more than the wife, as she kept saying how he always buys shit and then she has to sneak it in the trash. We had so much fun with them, but alas, they left without the furniture. Later that day, he showed up without her, laughing and said, "She may divorce me, but I want all of it." Chad and my dad, who couldn't get enough of him, told him they would even deliver it. I think he bought at least five pieces of furniture. I really hope she didn't divorce him after all their years of marriage.

After that, Mason House was pretty much empty and ready for demolition, but our work continued, especially on the yard. Mason House sits on an acre, an acre that hadn't been touched in probably thirty years. In the chaos of the overgrown property, the trees and plants were also more beautiful than any we'd ever seen. The azaleas were as big as a sedan, the Japanese maple was bigger than any we'd seen before, the rhododendrons were as tall as the house, but the brush we cleared seemed to never ever, ever end. We spent almost every evening and every weekend for four months working on the property while our contractors worked on the house and pool.

We created endless piles of brush cleaning up the land. We dug, we pulled, we sawed, we drug, and we came home at night sore, sweaty, bleeding and bit up. That part of the project felt like there was never an end in sight. We removed and cleaned up the big trees and pulled out terribly overgrown bushes in front of the house, completely changing the curbside appeal. We had a neighbor stop by just to thank us for cleaning up the front of the house. She told us how proud of us she was and how excited everyone was that we were saving the home instead of tearing it down to build a mansion. We chopped and chipped up endless branches; so many that I broke one of my fingers. We searched for buried treasure, never to be found…yet. We attempted to save some roses, azaleas and rhododendrons in hopes of planting them next year when we have an idea of what to do with this magnificent property.

While cleaning up the yard, we had some fun with the riding lawn mower Joan had left at the house and continued to dig through treasures left in the shed. On one of these days, Chad was working on the yard in Mason House while I was at our apartment taking care of the dogs when Joan stopped by. At this point, we hadn't heard anything from her in about four weeks. Joan told Chad that she knew she wasn't supposed to be there, but that she needed to renew her driver's license and needed to get into the black filing cabinet. The same cabinet she had emptied into a black garbage bag on her last day back in the house. Chad calmly explained to her that the house was empty; the contractors had already started and reminded her that she had already emptied the filing cabinet. She left quietly and without incident.

One of the bigger projects of the property was a huge tree smack in the middle of our back yard. The tree had been allowed to grow however it wished for the last fifty years. We assume the former owners had once run electric to it for Christmas lights. The lights and electric conduits were still there. They had also built a metal fence around it and never removed it. The tree was not only enormous and overgrown, but now there was literally metal grown into it. We had one tree removal bid that came in at $10,000. Ten thousand dollars to remove the huge metal monster tree! Our contractor found a guy who would take most of it down for about half of that, but it took him over two weeks and he was only willing to take it so far down due to the metal growing throughout. For months we had a gigantic stump in the middle of our yard. For a while, we really thought we'd be stuck with that damn stump and man, did people have suggestions as to what to have it carved into.

A lifeguard post for the pool.

A mermaid with big boobs, complete with blue crocheted nipple warmers.

A Totem pole.

A dog.

A table.

During this time, we also discovered they had also planted a beautifully fragrant garden of mint at the base of the tree.

We just wanted it gone. Finally, we found a guy from Southern Missouri who was willing to work on it. Amazingly, he whittled it down to the ground and readied it for sod. One hot afternoon while he and his crew chipped away at the monstrosity in our back yard, he flagged me down just to tell me that he was determined to conquer that damn tree for us!

A few weeks later, the Senior PGA was in town and all the houses along our street were allowing spectators to park in their front yards. It was a great way to spend a beautiful weekend outside, make some cash and get to know our new neighbors. It had already been quite a week for us. Earlier in the week, my friend Amanda called asking what the previous homeowner's last name was and told me she was pretty sure that we were on the news. The local Goodwill had spotted a shadowbox full of WWII medals that had, what they assumed, been accidently donated. Sure enough, they were from our house.

It ran on the front page of the Saint Louis Post Dispatch that next day, which just happened to be Memorial Day weekend.

I remembered the shadow box exactly. We had just gotten a call from our contractor saying our new dumpster was going to arrive within the next hour or so. Dumpsters cost over $300, so we needed to make sure we maximized it and filled it to the brim before they were switched out. Both of our parents were with us and we decided to tackle the seashell room to finish off the dumpster. What had been an additional master suite in the house had become a room that was so full that you couldn't walk into it at all. Behind all the junk, was an abstract wall of wood on one entire wall that Joan's mother had created using two-by-fours that she had cut into chunks, painted and glued to the wall. Additionally, she had plastered the ceiling with hundreds of seashells and mirrors in a mosaic pattern. It was one of the most strangely beautiful things we'd ever seen. With the dumpster deadline looming, all six of us started frantically emptying the room.

There was a mixed bag of everything in the seashell room, including mice. It was one of the dirtier rooms, and had the highest concentration of mice, dead or alive. This bedroom is where we found the brand new disco balls. This is also the room where there were no less than ten *Pier 1* bags full of Christmas candles and décor, never opened, but too damaged by mice bites or pee to either use or sell. This is also the room in which Chad's mom and mine moved a bag and a live mouse squealed and shot out and ran away. Actually, I think the squealing was mom and

Terry. The seashell room was home to the now famous shadowbox of WWII medals.

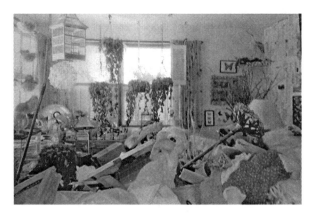

The full seashell room where
the WWII medals were found.

We quickly cleaned out the seashell room using the same system; donate, trash or keep and sell or refinish. I remember the shadowbox. I didn't think much about it, nor did I have the time to really look what was inside of it. I knew that there was no family left, so I thought to myself, "Well, Goodwill can at least sell the shadowbox." That is the only reason it didn't go directly into the dumpster.

Months later, Goodwill found the shadowbox filled with medals and contacted the media. The news story stated some of Joan's stepdad's history. He was a hero in WWII, a POW, truly an amazing story. The media was also trying to track down family, in which they were having no luck. Chad and I decided not to come forward. We didn't come forward then for a couple of reasons. For one, we didn't want to have to explain that the home was a hoarder house; it was not our place to name Joan as a hoarder publically. Secondly, I had made the mistake of reading the comments on the online version of the story and my fear was solidified; I didn't want to be portrayed as someone who doesn't appreciate history or the military. My brother-in-law is in the Air Force. I respect and love history. I had no idea how important or special those medals were. I just knew that I was in the midst of emptying an entire house in four days and the medals were a casualty of our hurried work.

We hoped the story would just run its course, but our friends and family kept sending us links to the story that had made its way across the country. The research behind it was phenomenal. Because I idiotically and accidently donated these medals, Goodwill had tracked down the war hero's biological daughter out in California. They had arranged to send them back to her. We were so thankful that at this point they were finally going to get to the right daughter. If I had stopped to think about those medals, we probably would have given them back to Joan, in which case, they would most likely just have been hoarded again. When the connection was made to the daughter in California, we decided to take one last look in the gross moldy basement. We had left a fair amount of items too damaged to do anything with to be trashed during demo of the house. In that last ditch effort, we found a box. A box that had gotten wet several times in the last thirty years and been used as a mice nest for the majority of them. Inside we found more history, a couple of his uniforms from his time in the Marines. They had his name stamped on the inside. They were in terrible shape, but they were a part of him. We figured we would hold onto them and somehow get them to the daughter.

That weekend, sitting outside attempting to make some cash while parking cars for the Senior PGA tournament, a car pulled into the driveway. Chad instantly looked at me and said, "Shit, I think that's the *Post Dispatch*. They found us." We had known that reporters had been by the house looking for the new owners while construction workers were demoing, but our names had not gone public yet. This wasn't the Post; it was a reporter from our local NBC affiliate.

"Are you the new owners of the home?" he asked us.

Chad and I looked at each other with scared apprehension.

"Yes."

The reporter told us he took the chance that we would be working on the property today and asked if we'd be willing to do an on camera spot for the newscast that night. Thank God, I at least put on some mascara and concealer that day! I told him he was going to be very pleased and would owe us, as there was a part of the story that hadn't gone public yet. We told him about the uniforms. We taped the segment and he promised to connect us with the people at Goodwill to make sure that everything would get to the daughter in California.

What we never told the newspaper or the news stations was that we had also found his funeral flag. I cleaned up the flags and uniforms as best as I could and gave them to the representative from Goodwill, who sent them off to the family in California along with the medals. I will never forget the phone call and the card we received from them thanking us for helping them preserve and put to rest the legacy of their family. It will always go down as one of the most heartwarming stories of Mason House.

The rest of the summer was spent checking on the progress of the construction on both the house and the pool. The pool construction was not only the most difficult, but also the most delayed. Chad and I checked on the property every night to see its' progress and make sure it was aligning with what we asked for. In less than ninety days, our home would be ready for move in. All that summer we were crammed in a small apartment with the three dogs, oftentimes hosting family and visitors when people came in town to help us work on the property. The best part of apartment living was all the baby ducks and geese that were born while we lived there. I was always the crazy woman seeing how close I could get to them to take pictures, feed and love on them.

Sure, there were some major frustrations in the construction process, the plumbing was done incorrectly and had to be re-done, the pool was delayed by over two months and was by far the most painful of the entire project due to frustrations and delays with permits, but overall, it was an amazing process. Before IVF, Chad and I never would have taken on a project like this. I wasn't a happy enough person and our marriage probably not strong enough. However, after surviving and eventually thriving after IVF we worked together as a strong unit. We never had any problems picking things out. Usually we agreed completely on it or one of us felt very strongly about it and the other one didn't care either way.

We saw Joan one more time, during a weekend we spent working on the property. Our contractor was at the house putting in the new cabinets and told us Joan had been at the house. She simply wandered the property aimlessly and would occasionally pick up pieces of wood and inspect them. She said hello to the contractors, blessed them and went on her way. I explained to our contractor that the next time they needed to call the police dispatch. Throughout the entire process, Joan was told that after the house sold she was not allowed back on the property and that if she did come, the police would be called. And we needed to stick to that plan, so I called dispatch and made a report. It was amazing, as soon as I stated our name and address, the police knew exactly what property we were referring to.

An officer came out and made up the report. He let us know that everyone on the force knows about Joan and although she's never been dangerous, we still need to be cautious. He also said that she probably slipped through the cracks all these years because she had never been dangerous. He told us to call next time she shows up and somebody will be there in a few minutes to deliver a verbal no trespassing warning and let her know that next time she would be arrested.

The next morning as we pulled up to the house, we saw Joan's car in our neighbor's driveway. We drove by to find that she was wandering around the backyard wearing kneepads with a plastic bag in her hands.

I immediately called dispatch who told us to circle the block and not scare her off, as officers were on the way. The same officer we spoke to the day before pulled up and we pulled in after him. The three of us started walking the property calling for Joan who was now hiding. The next thing I know, another police officer pulled in to block Joan's car in our neighbor's driveway. Then another came in and blocked off the main road. Finally, she answered us; she was hiding down in the creek behind house.

I was scared at this point. She's hiding in the back of the property from us. What is she doing here? What does she want? Why now, after a couple of months?

The officers brought her in front of us and explained to her that she could not come here ever again. The entire time she was mumbling that she knew she wasn't supposed to be here, that she had been told not to step onto the property. So she gets it, but she clearly wasn't absorbing anything anyone was saying. She then asked me for my phone number and again reminded me to keep Gertie, Gracie and Bosco off the main road. She remembered the dog's names! The officer from the day before was being extremely patient, but then again he had never really dealt with Joan face to face. They went through everything.

You can't come here to see what paint color they choose.

You can't come here to see what kind of air conditioner they put in.

You can't come here to dig up a root from the creek.

A sentence one never expects to hear from a police officer. She was literally in the creek on her hands and knees digging up a root. She was dazed in front of all of us, holding onto that root like it was the last thing she had left. I made eye contact with her, tears of fear filling my eyes. I'm not sure she ever really saw me though.

At this point the other officers were done. You could tell they had dealt with her before and they were done being nice. One yelled, "That's it, get off the fucking property. You aren't ever going to meet the dogs. Let's go!"

They led her to her vehicle and spent the next twenty minutes talking her off the property. Again, a report was made and we were told that the next time she would be arrested and they would like us to file official charges against her in the hopes that she would finally get help.

That was the last time we saw Joan. Although, I'm not sure I'll ever really feel positive that it will be the last time forever.

One of my favorite memories at Mason House to date was the day our pool was delivered. Fiberglass pools are all one piece, so the delivery day, much later than we had hoped, landed on a steamy August morning. Our parents, our friends and their kids whom we love so much came to see the pool craned over our new house. The pool people probably thought we were crazy; it's just a pool for goodness sake! The support we had was strangely amazing. But this pool is our baby in so many ways, and these people would never have missed its' delivery. We all watched with mouths wide open as the pool was craned upside down over Mason House and set in the backyard. Then it was lifted again to turn it right side up into the gigantic hole that would be our new pool. I will never forget the amazement on all of our faces and the sheer excitement and hope in the future memories that this pool would bring us all.

Throughout the entire process of emptying the house and working on the yard, we had so much help from family and friends, especially from our parents. They spent almost every weekend working on the yard, painting, or just plain helping. We will never be able to repay them and the only thing that comes even close are the memories we built that summer. Some of those memories took place when we were exhausted, very smelly and eating a late dinner at TGI Friday's. Friday's was two minutes from our apartment and they had an outdoor patio. We all probably should have been embarrassed by how rough we looked and how terrible we smelled, but we needed to eat, so we earned a lot of Friday's points that summer.

There is also no doubt in my heart and soul that we were able to get through the process because of all the help and support we received from our friends and family. There were plenty of people who would call us crazy to our face. And ask why. Why this house? Why a hoarder's house? Why? And to be honest, even now, I don't have the exact words. Only that it felt right. Mason house became our dream; it became our family, our children.

As we picked everything out and started to see everything come together, I could see our future. All the kids in our lives growing up with us, playing games in the basement with us, swimming in the pool every summer all summer long, this was it, Mason House was our future.

The love, support and connection that Mason House brought into our lives was remarkable. We will never forget the random people we met who simply stopped by to see the progress, or the people we met at several of the sales we held, and everyone who thanked us for saving the history of the house. The people who would come by who had some tie to the house because they had grown up somehow with the family before. The saving of Mason House brought us a sense that this was now going to be a home filled with happiness, love and laughter.

Mason House also brought so many people back into our lives. I chronicled the entire process on Facebook. I started at the very beginning with the shocking photos of the massive amounts of things the house contained. To the strange things we found inside, through the construction process, people followed, people prayed, people were entertained. Bottom line, people were drawn to it. Even if they didn't know our background or why we decided to move and remodel a hoarder house, they were still pulled to the story, our redefinition story.

I had friends reach out and want to help, after not seeing them for twelve years even. I had friends resurface, not after a falling out necessarily, but just because life got in the way. Mason House was this magnet for connection.

All our loved ones and friends, who saw us through IVF, again supported us through Mason House. Maybe never quite understanding what it was about this house, but knowing that this was our family now.

Mason House is our ever upward, in so many ways.

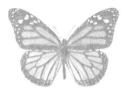

Chapter 8

Emerging to
Own Myself Again

other's Day 2013: On what would have been my first mother's day had IVF and surrogacy worked, I took the biggest leap of my life and sent out my first batch of query letters to publishers and agents. I had already begun to write this book as we were going through our IVF journey, only to lose it completely when my old, impatient and clumsy self, spilled water on my computer. Somewhere deep inside I've always known that I had a book inside of me even though I never considered myself a writer in any stretch of the word. When you spend your life, since the age of fourteen, with people asking how you survived living in a body cast for a year of your life, you know they are curious. I knew that I was built for survival. It was only after surviving failed IVF and surrogacy and fighting for my own recovery that I realized my story of not only survival but of how I now thrive was one that could help others and change lives. So, on what would have been my first Mother's Day, I took the risk of sending out my first batch of query letters for this book, *Ever Upward*. Then, I sat down and started writing it over. This time I made sure my water had a lid on it.

The work was slow; especially considering we were building our family home at Mason House. I also know I was allowing my shame and self-doubt to steal my light and my voice in completing the book, let alone in believing that anyone would actually want to read my story. I needed an inspirational kick in the pants, so I turned to Brené Brown. The work of Brené Brown had already changed so much of my life, but I knew there was more. That July, I started seeking a way in which I could maybe, just maybe, get to see Brené speak live, when I stumbled upon the Emerging Women conference. Emerging Women 2013 was scheduled for October in Boulder and the lineup of speakers was something only this therapist and someone fighting for recovery could dream up. It was a huge investment between the conference, flight and hotel accommodations and it would be so scary to go by myself, but something inside of me just knew I needed to be there. So I talked it over with Chad, stated my case to him, both as my husband and JBF Therapy & Coaching's accountant. Looking back, I know I was also convincing myself that I needed to be in Boulder that October, and that I deserved to be there.

I arrived at the beautiful St. Julien Hotel in Boulder, CO on a cool Thursday evening in October. I had clients to see that morning, so I had to miss some of the Power Circle activities from that afternoon, but I was able to make it in time for what I knew would be my most important keynote speaker that night, Brené Brown. I was much more anxious than I thought I would be. I didn't know anyone there. It seemed like every other woman had come with a friend or colleague. I got my dinner plate and then looked out into a sea of women of every age. The anxious excitement was palpable, and wasn't only coming from me, making my heart race and my palms sweat. I simply sat down at my assigned table and started introducing myself. I was surprised at how few people had heard of Brené, since she was the main reason I was there. As we moved into the venue for Brené's talk, I could feel my anxiety slowly replaced with excited light. Upon spotting Brené sitting next to and laughing with Elizabeth Gilbert, author of *Eat, Pray, Love* that excited light turned into giddy, schoolgirl heart fluttering. These were *my* famous people. The women whose books and research I absorbed throughout the years like a sponge. The women who have helped me change my life so many times over. This was going to be an amazing few days.

Brené's talk was just as fulfilling as I expected it to be. I waited in line for an hour and half for her signature in my *The Gifts of Imperfection* book. This is where I met a couple of women I would spend the next few days getting to know better and build friendships that would carry us throughout the future. I was about twenty people away from getting to say, "Hello" to one of my idols, when they closed the line because Brené had to catch a flight home. Disappointed, I walked away knowing that I would see her in February, as I had already applied and been accepted to her Daring Way™ certification training for helping professionals. I went to bed that night both exhaustedly fulfilled and so eager for the next day's events.

The next day was full, with keynote speakers and two workshops of my choosing. The anxiety washed away as I embraced and allowed all the pure light to wash over me while I took a deep breath knowing that I was exactly where I was meant to be. I received a message I needed to hear from every speaker at Emerging Women. I ferociously took notes and soaked up the knowledge, energy and the undeniable spark that something great was at work, both within myself, and between all of these amazing women. My first huge a-ha moment was during the keynote speech of Elizabeth Gilbert, author of *Eat, Pray, Love*. She spoke to us about what she called the shameless pursuit of magic. She told us the story of how she came to write and eventually publish her most recent fiction novel, *The Signature of All Things*. She spoke on how she had some concept of the book three different times; to only then lose it somehow. She said magic will roam about this earth looking for its mother asking, "Are you my mother?"

"Are you my mother?"

"Are you my mother?"

Until magic finds its mother.

As I listened to Elizabeth speak those words and tell her truth of letting go of her first three tries at her now very successful novel in order to embrace her real work, I felt my heart skip a beat. I had to lose those three babies in order to find my path, to follow my magic. This was that very first spark of knowing that Ever Upward was it. My magic had found its mother.

Next up was the first workshop of my choice with Kelly McGonigal, author *of The Willpower Instinct*. With Kelly, we worked on creating the change we wanted to see in our lives. The most striking lesson from this workshop for me was in being honest with myself as to why I wanted to publish my story in Ever Upward. Kelly took us through our ego-system versus eco-system reasons for creating the change. Ego-system reasons are for ourselves or revolve around us, our egos. Eco-system reasons are about care for others, connection and interdependence. It was within this work that I was honest about the obvious ego reasons, but for the first time I really saw my eco reasons. They are the reasons that I do this work, live this life and do it all out loud. I wrote this book to own that a childfree is okay, to create conversation and open empathy to infertility, to connect with others, and to help others. If I am completely honest with myself, these are some of the exact same reasons that drove me to be a therapist and will continue to drive my future projects; it is the core of who I am.

Kelly also had us write a letter from our future selves. As I write this last chapter of Ever Upward, I reread the letter I wrote to myself six months ago and am filled with peace.

> "Dear Justine,
>
> I'm so happy and proud of you for the work you did, and are continuing to do, to allow yourself and push yourself to finish Ever Upward and get published. Your braveness to complete it from a place of authenticity and connection rather than as proof was phenomenal. I am proud of the commitment and sacrifices you made to complete the publishing process, but more importantly to complete the book. You've been able to change everything and will find that the work is amazingly worth it, in relationships and connection and peace. Most of all, I'm proud that you had the courage to let go of defensiveness, attention, admiration in order to embrace connection and love.
>
> Ever Upward to Dare Greatly with Brave Courage, Justine"

That night, we were assigned to small dinner groups with the speakers from the conference. My group was paired with Erin Weed, Founder of Girls Fight Back and thought leader at Evoso. She asked us each to talk about what brought us to Emerging Women and what we were focusing on throughout the conference. I, of course, was honest about Brené being the original reason I registered and then I spoke about getting Ever Upward published with the short version of back surgeries, IVF and my now childfree life. Erin looked me dead in the eyes and told me that she could tell I am a therapist who is knowledgeable in the research, but she needed me to go beyond Brené's work and words. She said, "You have your own epic story to tell, give me your words!" Right then and there, all eyes on me, I stumbled a bit with "embrace, solidify, grow…" my voice shaking and palms sweating. Finally, with that all too familiar deep knowing breath, I opened my mouth and said; "I will own and not just prove."

It was with these words, "own and not just prove," that I felt my calling, my purpose. I needed to own every single part of my story and not just prove it. I needed to stop trying to prove that my path is okay. That not doing another round of IVF is okay. That not being a mother is okay. That not adopting is okay. Stop trying to prove it and just own it. Own my struggles in the IVF world. Own that I stopped treatments. Own that I don't want to adopt. Own that I am more than childless. Own that I will practice and fight for my recovery and own my childfree life. The first full day of training was the push I needed to find my voice again. To finally find my light.

Day Two began with Kristen Wheeler, a consultant and coach, who spoke about finding and living our Native Genius™. She spoke about our innate desires and tuning in to and being amazed by what is automatic in us. She calls this Native Genius™. What is something you love to do? Do you feel your purpose, your calling in doing it? You can't not do it? This, according to Kristen Wheeler, is our Native Genius™. I felt like I had a sense of what my purpose was, especially after day one, but something I carried home with me from Kristen's speech was to add this question to my nighttime journal every night. I wasn't surprised in the least when for the next year, my Native Genius™ was always working with clients or writing.

I had the honor of seeing Kristin Neff, self-compassion researcher, speak twice that day on learning how we all must open our hearts to ourselves in order to truly do it with anyone else. I came completely prepared to learn with several of my clients in mind, to her workshop on self-compassion. Well, the universe will always conspire for you. I learned Neff's Self-Compassion Break meditation in that training and lo and behold, it was for me. I realized how I berate myself every day about the very things that probably make me, well, me. I also learned how to turn this around some and make these traits work more for me rather than against me through validation and self-kindness. Day Two also included one of the most powerful hours of my life. Eve Ensler, author of the *Vagina Monologues,* read from her new book, *In the Body of the World* and spoke of the healing power of connection; connection to ourselves, our bodies, each other and the earth. Women were left in their seats sobbing, both with the rawness of identification but also with the completed wholeness within one another and ourselves.

That evening, I received a Facebook message from a sorority sister from college. She and her husband were staying at the same hotel for his boss' birthday. They knew I had as busy a schedule as they did, but she really wanted to meet up for a glass of wine that evening. So, before heading to the Emerging Women private Ani DiFranco concert, which was unbelievable by the way, I met up with Ashley and Matt for a glass of red wine and what ended up being my permission slip for Ever Upward.

Ashley and I weren't necessarily in the same group in college and as life often happens, we weren't connected in our adult lives. We had seen each other a few times at Ranken Jordan Pediatric Bridge Hospital events (where I volunteer in the nursery holding and rocking babies) and caught up some. Last time, I had filled her in on our whole kids situation. Then she finally joined and became active on Facebook and our connection sparked. It doesn't hurt that she has always been one of the nicest and most positive people and her children are some of the cutest on my Facebook wall, so I am always commenting on them. We sat and caught up for a bit, I filled Matt in on what the conference was all about and then she shooed him away to get our drinks. Ashley then proceeded to thank me. She said how much knowing my story, my courage to share it and to even post an article about infertility on Facebook has helped her to understand more about the struggles of infertility, especially as a blessed mom of three beautiful children. She said my vulnerability and truth have made her a better friend and person. And with that, the purpose I felt the day before was solidified.

I smiled with goose bumps and tears and muttered the words, "thank you." She just gave me the permission, the nudge I needed, to know that my story needed to be heard.

I spent the last day of the Emerging Women Conference listening to amazing speakers with souls I cherish like Alanis Morissette and Tami Simon. Both women emulated the message of finding your soul's purpose, sitting with it, owning it and then finding your way for the world to see it. I felt like I needed a week off to let everything and everyone soak in. The speakers, the energy and the fellow women literally helped me to find my spark and to finally own it. I can't say what made me fight for and figure out how to get to Emerging Women, I just knew I had to be there. It was one of the most powerful experiences I've ever had in reclaiming me.

I am also immensely thankful for the women I met at Emerging Women. Sarah my quirky artsy friend with the funky glasses I so wanted for myself, who now works for Emerging Women. Erica, who I laughed with and learned so much from and who helped me so much with finding the focus for this very book. Tanya, who's amazing story of survival felt like seeing my own light in her. Sarah and Marie, the mother and daughter, I met with and connected with so much on the cab ride on the very first day; seeing them together, their friendship, gave me permission to find my purpose in *Ever Upward* in ways I am not quite able to explain. Tova, my early morning breakfast buddy and someone who knew the strength required for survival. Melinda, my fellow Brené fan and also a childfree woman. And Michele, a soul sister who I saw so much of myself in, especially in our professional selves.

I came home and really began to finish this very book.

Three short weeks later, after researching what it takes to get published, I started Ever Upward the blog.

In my very first post of "Ever Upward" (blog), I was honest with my intentions. I started it to build credibility with agents and publishers for the eventual publishing of *Ever Upward* the book, I started it as part of my healing journey and I started it because I knew the world needed my voice and I wanted to help and connect with others like me.

The blogging world is full of infertility bloggers. I know this because I sought out support and refuge in them while Chad and I were going through our own journey. However, on this side of recovery I found these blogs to be missing what I needed. Many of them chronicled their IVF treatments, their numbers of measurements in medications and vaginal ultrasounds. They were filled with follicle counts, Clomid crazy train side effects and awful recounts of painful medical procedures. They were women who were still deep in the throes of treatment. Then there were the bloggers who wrote about when the treatments finally worked or when the adoption finally went through. Once again, I was faced with the hard fact that I just didn't fit in. Fortunately, through my work on my own recovery I knew this didn't mean that "Ever Upward" (blog) didn't belong.

It wasn't long before I knew there was something special both in me and in this blog, something bigger than I may ever get the honor of knowing. I was able to write my soul. I was able to write my light, without much apology. The need for my further healing, for owning my shame, and the need to give voice to this side of fertility fueled me forward. The days I didn't write, I struggled. Chad turned to me one day and said, "I can tell the days you aren't writing." This healing through the authentic truth, help and connection is something that is almost indescribable.

I made connections with people from all over the world. I met a woman who had lost two sets of twins, both sets stillborn. We supported one another in our very different places of recovery, me accepting a childfree life and her waiting for the go ahead to start trying again. I met a couple of women who were just taking their first steps to end IVF treatments and figure out how they could possibly move forward to accept a childfree life. I met a never-to-be father struggling with the decision of whether or not he and his wife wanted to move forward with the process of adoption.

Then I found Marie. "Ever Upward" is tiny, especially in the beginning, compared to Marie's blog, "Journeying Beyond Breast Cancer." Not only has she been viewed over 800,000 times, but she has also won awards, such as The Top Cancer Blog and Most Inspiring Health Blog. Every week Marie posts a Weekly Round Up of her favorite readings for the week. I took the chance and commented on it, thanking her for the work she puts into that post each week and asking her to take a look at my most recent post. Not only did she read and comment on my tiny little blog, but also we forged an unlikely friendship. Marie found some of herself in my story, as I have found a lot of myself in hers. She introduced "Ever Upward" to her many followers and other breast cancer bloggers because sadly, a lot of them have the whole infertility and childfree living in common. I am continually grateful and honored that she frequently includes my posts in her Weekly Round Ups. But, I am even more thankful for the understanding, the 'I get you' friend I have found in her. One day, we will meet, hopefully in her home country of Ireland.

Within the first six months of the conception of "Ever Upward" the blog, I wrote a few guest posts for other websites and bloggers and I posted myself at least a couple of times per week. I post about infertility and my story but mostly I post about life and recovery. There are some posts I have been scared to death to write, let alone hit the publish key, then there have been those that were so easy to publish that it felt like I couldn't breathe until I did.

The power of "Ever Upward" has been in the connections, not in the view counts or the number of shares, although I will readily admit how validating all of that feels. The real power is in how many people take the time to share my posts and add their comments of gratitude or compliment, or the hundreds of messages, through either the blog or privately, that I've received. These posts come from total strangers across the globe, from people I've haven't heard from in a long time and even from my everyday friends and family. The most power is when I can observe my courage being actively contagious. Including when my good friend Sam forwarded me a message she had received on Facebook from an old school friend of hers. The message said that the woman was in bed feeling sorry for herself after her sixth egg retrieval when she stumbled upon "Ever Upward" because Sam had shared it on her wall. She thanked her for the inspiration and for the understanding and the permission to own the fact that she struggles with infertility. The next day Sam called to tell me this woman posted on her Facebook wall that she had decided to start an infertility support group at her church. Without any words powerful enough and tears in my eyes, I took a deep knowing breath and felt my purpose and soaked in my ever upward.

I feel my purpose when my friend Kelly, my oldest friend, my friend who took care of me in a body cast and the friend who has come back into my life, shares every single blog post on Facebook. Every. Single. Post. Then one day, she shared with a comment of how she and her husband have had to use assisted fertility treatments for the first time publicly.

Both my biggest life lesson and the thing that has brought me the most amazing fulfillment through "Ever Upward" is discovering just how powerful courage is. If owning my shame, owning my story and speaking all the parts of it out loud, even the really scary parts, inspires one single person to own their story, well, then it is completely worth every word of judgment and misunderstanding I've struggled with.

It has been a constant struggle for me to balance my desire for "Ever Upward" to get noticed and have astronomical numbers, not only for personal validation, but also for the bigger purpose of helping others, with the all-knowing sense that as long as it helps just one person own their story and fight for their recovery, then it is worth it.

I started "Ever Upward" for publishing credit. I continue to write "Ever Upward" because of the connections I have made with people from all over the world and with very different stories than mine that are surprisingly the same. I don't know if I will ever be noticed by the editors at WordPress to be Freshly Pressed, or if Huffington Post will ever pick up one of my posts to run or if I will ever have hundreds of thousands of followers, but I do know that I will continue writing. I will write for myself, for my healing and for everyone else who finds my tiny spark just the spark they need to start choosing their own recovery, to choose themselves again and to find their own courage.

The 2013 holidays felt so different from previous years. A decent amount of time had passed since ending our IVF journey and we were coming up on the last never to be first birthday on December 21, 2013. This was our first holiday season in Mason House. It was also our first holiday season completely off the IVF roller coaster. No two week wait of hoping for a positive pregnancy test and the first holiday season without the sadness of the never to be due date. Our first holiday season after spending the last year rebuilding ourselves, grieving our losses, accepting our story and redefining us. I was feeling much better, finding my footing again as a human, as a woman, as a childfree woman. I was finding me again. Chad and I sat down and talked about what we really wanted our holidays to be like and to figure out what our traditions were going to be now that this was us, a childfree couple; it was time to do what I truly do best, redefine.

Redefining meant picking out our very first real Christmas tree. We were some of the first ones at the lot that night and much like everything

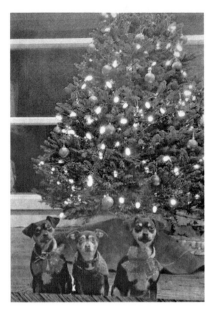

Christmas redefined.

we picked with Mason House, it took just minutes to find our perfect tree. With that first real Christmas tree, a tree that smelled so delicious that I actually tried to hug it, our holiday traditions were born! Thanksgiving eve includes picking out our tree, getting Mexican food for dinner, having a margarita, decorating the tree and taking a hundred pictures of the dogs to get just one good one.

Thanksgiving tends to be our busiest holiday because we cram in both sides of our family in three short days. This year, we decided to add something just for us. We made a deal that one of our holiday traditions would be to go see a movie, just the two of us, on Thanksgiving night, after leaving Chad's family at his aunt's house. This first year, I was very thankful for that plan. That day, at Thanksgiving lunch with his family, we had an unexpected surprise that I was not prepared for. There was a baby at lunch whose parents were teenagers and whose name was Mason, which was our boy name (I know, the fact that we now have a house on Mason road is amazingly ironic). We are unsure, but the timing seems to work out, that this baby was also the baby that Chad's relatives had previously asked us to adopt. I wasn't warned, and maybe it wasn't even that baby, but it hit me like a two-ton shield and left me standing there with my heart pounding, body sweating, and hands shaking. Chad looked at me and mouthed, "Go to the bathroom." I cried, pulled myself together and got through the day. It hurt, it was unexpected and it felt like a huge slap in the face, but I knew we had our traditions to look forward to that night.

That night, I was very upset at home and tried to explain why I was so upset to Chad, but all I could come up with was that I should have been told about it and that it was again, just one of those slaps in the face: why the hell don't we get to have kids!?

I love children, I love when my loved ones get to have children; I even love when strangers, hell, people I don't even like, get to have children. Where I struggle is with the people who "don't deserve" them: the super fertile 16 year olds, the couple who have already lost custody of their other three children, or the people who really don't want them. I'm sure this list could go on and on, just watch the news. No emotion is uncomplicated for a therapist. This brief, but very strong, bitter angry emotion knocks me down momentarily, but as I continue to do the work to redefine myself, I am learning to rebound more quickly. I am also learning to understand more about myself, and how I feel about the "don't deserves."

1. I am NO ONE to judge who gets the joy of children. I am neither judge nor jury, nor do I want to be.
2. I do have faith that there are no mistakes, at least in the long run.
3. Even though it feels really, really, freaking unfair, it really is neither fair nor unfair. Sure, maybe it's unlucky, but it just is, and it is not necessarily mine to understand.
4. Most importantly, I am coming to understand that this anger is coming in to save me from feeling what I really feel… which is simply really sad.

And, that is okay, sometimes things are just sad. It's sad that IVF didn't work for us. It's sad that we lost our three babies. It's sad that we lost those three dreams. Giving myself permission to continue to feel that sadness, as needed, will help to stave off that anger that seems to set me back in my recovery so much every time. I have to embrace it in order to let it go. When I allow myself to feel it, I don't become it. Only when I do this, is there enough space to find the ever upward. The ever upward that is this work of learning to be happy and healthy, and even okay and fulfilled, without children. We all must work to accept that we are not wired to escape ourselves, no matter how hard we try. We have to feel, we have to feel it all, even the darkness, because when we allow ourselves to do that, it will pass and make room for the light.

One holiday down, Christmas left to go, but first, the last never to be first birthday. I am sure that to many people, they were only eight cell embryos of Chad and I implanted into Michelle's uterus, never to complete gestation. But to us, they were our babies, our future dreams, and that last never to come true dream was due on December 21st, 2012. On December 21st, 2013, we marked our last never to be first birthday, and with it I felt the universe; sad, mad and bitter, but more than that I felt happy, content and peaceful. I felt a sense that everything was as it was supposed to be in my universe. I felt that peaceful and yet bittersweet pull of my soul. It was that day that I was able to truly claim my ongoing, thriving acceptance.

My ongoing, thriving acceptance means I wear a mother's ring and necklace with what would have been the birthstones of our never to be children. If you ask me if they are my kids or if they are the birthstones of my dogs, I will not shy away from your questions. I will own my truth.

I will tell you that we tried to have children; we tried really hard, with lots of money, pain and love, but it was never our dream to have.

I will tell you they were my children, never to be mine on this physical earth.

I will tell you that I am an ever evolving, and sometimes not so pretty, work in progress in accepting my childfree life.

And, I will tell you that December 21ˢᵗ, 2013, that day, more than ever, I became sure that my journey through IVF, that those three babies are...

My completion.

My sorrowful joys.

My lights.

My ever upward.

Many childless couples choose to travel during the holiday season. They get out of town and enjoy the sunshine on a beach or go hit the slopes somewhere far away from the holiday crowds and all the traditions that revolve around children. Perhaps there will be a day when Chad and I are drawn to this way of spending the holiday season, but for now, I'm still not quite ready to miss out on being a part of the childlike wonder and magic of Christmas.

Christmas 2013 started in a very unusual way for us. I had this strong need to attend the Christmas Eve service (my first ever) at a new church my colleague had been trying to get me to attend for a while. For the first time, in forever, I felt at peace in a church setting; the music was beautiful and the message powerful and I finally didn't feel so alone.

Coming in to that holiday season, Chad and I were constantly reminded of this sense of feeling alone as a childless couple. After a particularly difficult weekend, of me feeling a strong sense of not fitting in anywhere as a 30 something year old woman without any kids, Chad came up with a brilliant idea for a new Christmas tradition with our friends' children. We began the tradition of having our own little Christmas celebrations with our closest friends and their boys (all of our close friends have three boys). Each year we will buy three gifts for each family that the boys must share: a gift to take home, a gift to keep at our house to play with, and a Wii game for them to play when they visit us. Each year, we will have the families join us for dinner, and our own little

Christmas gift opening party. This way Chad and I still get a tiny piece of the childlike wonder of Christmas.

This year, we also began the tradition of making rounds on Christmas day to see what Santa brought all the boys. This was one of my favorite memories growing up. We would go to all of our cousins' houses to see what Santa brought them. Later, when they were out and about making the rounds, they would come to our house so we could have our own show and tell. This first year my parents were here with us, so they also got to make the rounds with us. It really was a special memory for us all to see the boys describe what Santa brought them and play with their new toys.

Making my own Christmas magic within my childfree life also means we get to have some adult fun during the holidays. This was our first Christmas in Mason House and starting our family traditions in our forever family home. We were able to have family stay with us, cook yummy meals, drink scrumptious wine and play charades with our family. I didn't have to watch my sailor potty mouth or be nervous about the dogs and children. There can be ever upward magic within this adult Christmas too.

Ending IVF and living a childfree life means lifelong losses. The Christmas season seems to highlight these losses so much that sometimes it can feel like I am a gaping, oozing wound. I will never get to be Santa for my own children. I will never get to see their eyes and face light up with pure, joyful magic as they talk about Santa Claus or leave cookies out for him on Christmas Eve. I will never watch them in the Christmas play or sing in the holiday concert. But, I can still make my own magic to find my ever upward, and I hope that everyone else can stop and take a moment to feel the magical love that Christmas gives us all. Stop, take a breath and be grateful for your version of holiday magic. My magic, the magic of our childfree lives, will include all the child*full* Christmas traditions, and otherwise, that we chose to begin the season of 2013, because, after all, choosing joy, and magic, is a choice.

Getting through our first holiday season as a true childfree couple left us with a stronger marriage. It also found me continuing the ever upward journey of my recovery. In February of 2014, I left for San Antonio for five days of training with Brené Brown and her team for The Daring Way™ certification. It was a huge investment, financially and time wise. I was anxious because I would not know any other professionals there but also because I knew I was embarking on something great.

Our training was on the beautiful San Antonio Riverwalk. The hotel was stunning, the food was fabulous, the other women were amazing and the work was difficult and scary! Brené herself trained us in a large group, consisting of about 160 men and women, on the first day. For the next three days, we were split into rooms that consisted of our medium group (about twenty women) and a further split into a smaller group (nine women in mine). During those three days, we went through The Daring Way™ curriculum, both as a client and as students learning to facilitate the material. They were three of the most exhausting, but exhilarating, days of my life.

As a client works through The Daring Way™ curriculum, they are asked to keep one lens in mind, one arena. It could be their recovery, their relationships, their work, etc. For training purposes, we were asked to keep ours professional. Many of the women were focusing on marketing themselves better, building a strong private practice, getting started back up in private practice, etc. Without a doubt, I knew my focus throughout the work needed to be a little different, as I already had a successful practice, a great website and wrote for local publications. However, I needed to get ready to own my story and the part of my career that would be the blog finally gaining recognition and the eventual publishing of this very book. My small group was amazing enough to allow me to work through this arena.

Throughout The Daring Way™ work, I learned so much about what was really holding me back. I learned about my biggest shame triggers, and my wanted and unwanted identities when it comes to owning this part of my story. I was able to verbalize that I was fearful of being seen as selfish because I knew adoption was not our path. I was afraid of being thought of as not good enough of a therapist since I wasn't adopting. I was afraid of being seen as too messed up, or not healed enough, to be the great therapist I am. I learned that I was putting what I thought others might think of me, ahead of owning my own story, of owning me!

It was also through this work that I felt a direct connection to my back surgeries. I figured out that when I am around others, especially mothers, I tend to shut down my story. I ask them a lot about their lives and about their families, then I shut down because I assume I know what I will get from them when they discover I can't have kids. More times than not, it's sympathy and the need of the other person to take away my pain, which leaves me feeling invalidated and invisible, exactly how I felt when I was stuck in a body cast.

I had so much help during my back surgeries and I had amazing friends and family spend a lot of time with me, but no one could ever really get what I was going through. They all just had a lot of sympathy, really pity, for me; and I can't blame them, it must have felt so impossible for someone to empathize with me at the ages of 14 and 17, stuck in a body cast and missing school. Ultimately, their pity just meant that I felt even more alone, so I sucked it up – "chin up," as my dad always says, and in doing so, I snuffed out my light. It is only now that I have realized that my recovery from infertility, IVF and accepting a childfree life is what needed to happen for me to find my light again.

When people learn that you can't have kids, they feel bad for you. They feel sad for you. They want to fix it and take away the pain, which only makes me feel even more alone. Through my work with The Daring Way™, I am learning never to back down from my story, no matter how uncomfortable or sad it may make someone feel, because really, it is only through this emotional connection that anyone will truly see me and understand.

Just like at Emerging Women, I met some amazing friends at The Daring Way™ certification training, friends who are spread all over Northern America. They are friendships forged quickly through our shame work together. They are friends who provided amazing opportunities for me to use my voice, especially in regards to the arena I was focusing on.

Nicole was newly pregnant, and so sick with all day "morning" sickness. We were able to talk openly about what it is like for me to be around someone newly pregnant. She flat out asked me if it was hard. I will always treasure this honesty from her because it gave me the opportunity to use my voice. I was genuinely happy for her and I was able to admit that my biggest struggle is with people who I deem "undeserving" of having children and how much I battle with letting this anger go. Sabrina who also struggled with infertility for years before her and her husband adopted, in her I felt my fellow warrior light. Jen who thinks she wants children, but at the age of thirty-eight knows that infertility treatments may be her only option. Melissa who at one point said how bad she felt when she complained about how difficult it is being a working mom in front of me, someone who cannot have children. These women all provided me with the opportunity to do the work I needed to do to practice my shame resilience skills and to truly to own all the parts of my story. We also forged forward from difficult work to create undoubtedly lifelong, albeit long distance, friendships.

It wasn't much after The Daring Way™ training when I was due for my Lunch and Learn presentation at a local corporation here in Saint Louis. It was my sixth Lunch and Learn with them. I have always had good attendance, great feedback and they actually pay me to speak.

And yet that morning, even though I was over-prepared, I literally made myself sick with anxiety and self doubt. Because, that day I spoke on Wholehearted Parenting.

And, I am not a parent.

And, I was scared to death.

A few days before the presentation my shame consumed me as the presentation got closer; "I am not a parent and I am speaking on parenting." I remind myself that this is also major public information now through my blog. The self-doubt settled over me like a thick fog casting fear inside my very core.

Shame.

Horrible, suffocating shame.

Like the dementor to my light, stealing my voice, sucking away my soul, leaving my heart empty.

I reached out to my friend, Janine, who organizes the talks and she of course gave me an amazing pep talk. And then the night before the presentation my friend and colleague, Kelly, reminded me that I *am* actually a parent. Kelly's words will forever and always mean the world to me. She said I parent as much as she does to her two sons, just in different ways; I parent my dogs and I parent all of the children in my life and that most of all, I parent my clients. In many ways therapy is like parenting or even re-parenting with clients. She parents her two boys, but my audience of children is simply bigger as this is my purpose and my path.

I cried and took in her words because I knew they were my truth. I drew in that familiar deep knowing breath and thanked her for reminding me of my light. She reminded me of what I know every day in many ways, I wasn't given the chance or blessing of my own children because I am meant for this greatness of working with clients, writing and helping others. It's neither better nor worse or more or less important, it's just different.

So, that morning before I walked into that board room I wrote myself a permission slip, just like we ask ourselves and clients to do as they work through The Daring Way™ curriculum. I wrote myself my permission slip and set it right beside my notes.

"I have permission to be scared. I have permission to not be parent enough. I have permission to know, and own, that I know what I am talking about and that I can help even though I am not a parent in the traditional sense."

And so I spoke. And I was painfully vulnerable in owning to them that I am not a parent but that I was there to teach them about wholehearted parenting. I called out my own imposter syndrome, and let them in to my world: I don't get to be a parent but I think I can still help you be a better one. I also stated that I am the right person to do that because, one, I actually have the time to read the research and parenting books because I wasn't able to be a mom. And two, I parent every single day, just not my own children (and according to Kelly this probably means my house is cleaner, I am better rested and I have more sex).

I was real, I was vulnerable and I allowed my brilliant light to outshine my shame. And because I fought for that bravery, I connected and delivered one of my best lectures. And I have no doubt that there will be some families with some new language and new ways to love and parent because of that hour we spent together that day.

Between Emerging Women, The Daring Way™, my improved friendships all around and how much I changed in this year of my recovery I thought I had had a grasp on things. I sure as hell never thought I would feel the need to put anything about faith in *Ever Upward*. But, here I am, grappling with something new, changing myself, and of course, doubting things a lot. So, in other words, I must write about it.

I will easily admit that I have not ever had the strongest religion in my life. However, I have had something that can surely be considered some type of faith. Chad and I began regularly attending our new church since that Christmas Eve service. The pastor had begun a sermon series on the book of James, a fourteen-week long sermon series in fact. The first sermon included the passage, "Consider it pure joy..." Meaning, everything that happens to us, but especially the difficult times, are there to build perseverance and that we must shift our perspective to consider it pure joy.

Ever upward...

I have been stumbling along this path with my faith ever since.

"Hold it all together
Everybody needs you strong
But life hits you out of nowhere
And barely leaves you holding on
...You're not alone, stop holding on and just be held
Your world's not falling apart, it's falling into place..."

These are the lyrics to the song "Just Be Held" by Casting Crowns, that a friend posted on Facebook during a week I really needed it, Sure, it is a Christian band and song, but I dare you to listen to some of the lyrics and see if they can apply to your life, even if Christianity isn't your path.

I think we have to believe in something; having faith in something is a requirement of surviving this life, let alone thriving through recovery. As I work with my clients, I don't really care what they have faith in; God, Mother Nature, Karma, Life, Family, Relationships, Science, Coffee or that Pencil sitting on their desk. Life is too hard, especially in the really hard, messy times, not to have faith in something outside of ourselves, to believe in something or someone bigger than ourselves, to know that we are always understood and never alone.

I have spent most of my adult life struggling with religion while maintaining a decent amount of my own faith. Because frankly, there is nothing like being a mental health therapist who has struggled with infertility to make one doubt faith, a higher power, and especially, organized religion at times. However, within this doubt I never stopped searching. It has been through my recovery and what has felt like a never-ending search that I felt like I have finally found my home in faith and in religion. I cannot not write about faith when I share about my recovery, I guess, I just wish for all of us fighting the fight of recovery to seek something in the faith department. Seek something outside of yourself. Seek something bigger than you are, because within that search you may just finally find yourself again. You may just find your own ever upward.

What I am continuing to figure out about this life, about this recovery, about this redefinition of life after infertility is that there is only so much in my power to make better. I am continuing to figure out that as long as I do the work, and practice, to not just prove this is all okay and that I am okay, I make the room to really own it. When I do this work, the why's aren't so suffocating.

How do we sit with the be all, end all questions, what is this all supposed to mean? Why did this happen?

Aren't we all wondering the why?

Why does the 35-year-old mother of two young children get late stage colorectal cancer?

Why did he cheat?

Why did she have to die?

Why did he have to fall?

Why did they leave?

Why didn't I die?

Why are they lying?

Why did this have to happen???

Why?

But, I'm not sure we will ever get to know the why.

And, what I think I am learning is that some of our answers can be found in our almost enough moments.

You know those moments where you look up (to who or whatever you believe in, for me it is God) and say, "Okay, I get it. I would not have this if that had all worked out. Or, I would not have this if I had not lost that." But really, that just doesn't feel like it's quite enough? So, we question it; *I get it, I'm thankful, but it's still not enough for all that pain, all that suffering, the never-to-be's; I sure hope you have more, better, in the works.* I am learning we all have to figure out how to open ourselves up to these almost enough moments, really embracing their capacity for awe.

Can I have the presence and gratitude to embrace that piece of almost enough? Can I have faith that I might get to see the pieces all fit together one day? Better yet, can I have the presence and gratitude, and *patience*, enough to have the faith that I just may not get to see them all fit together and that the almost enough is, well, enough?

Because without a doubt, I have some pretty amazing almost enough moments of my infertility losses and childfree life...

Being McKinley's godparents.

Being asked to be in the delivery room to help bring baby Smith into this world.

Every moment with our chosen children.

Attending the piano recitals, church concerts and ball games of all our chosen children.

My friends through Emerging Women, The Daring Way™ certification and the Ever Upward blog.

Our Christmas morning tradition of going to see what Santa brought our chosen children.

The healing journey of writing this book.

A better marriage.

Building our family home, Mason house, for all our friends and family to grow and enjoy with us.

The continuing journey of my blog.

Becoming a better therapist.

Our dogs.

My improved relationships.

The happier, healthier me.

Fighting for me, fighting for my recovery and rediscovering my light.

I could go on and on, because I am able to wholeheartedly say that the list of my almost enough moments truly is endless.

My soul will always have the scars of our three lost babies, of three lost dreams, of three never-to-be's. Only I can choose to accept this as my whole story and move forward, having the faith that everything is exactly as it is supposed to be, no matter the why. Will I trust and have enough patience to know that these almost enough moments will lead me to understanding that my suffering, better yet, my story, will end exactly as it is meant to? Can I learn to have enough patience and faith to know that I might never get that final moment of completion, understanding and the good enough reason for my sufferings. Instead, I must figure out a way to be okay with that. I must learn to be whole without those enough moments. Trusting that the sole purpose I think I have found is only my plan, and I'm not sure I really get that much say in it.

I also have to learn to keep that in check with the part of me that yearns for my losses to mean something bigger, to change the world and help others. The part of me that asks, why else would I have been given this path in life? Why else would I have suffered the way I have and lost what I have? What would the point be of that? Am I that undeserving? Or, is this my punishment for something? Surely, it has to mean something; two back surgeries, a year in a body cast, two rounds of failed IVF with a surrogate, three lost babies and fighting for recovery can't just be it, can it?

And there it is again... Why did this have to happen to me?

I am not sure these questions come from the best part of me. However, I also know I wouldn't be honoring myself if I didn't allow this doubt a space to question; and maybe that is exactly the point.

We are only capable of understanding so much in this life, and maybe we're only allowed to understand so much. Maybe I will always have to create this constant balance between finding my purpose through my story of struggle, making sure it means something more, at least to me, and trusting that it will still mean just as much without the soul-completing clarity I so desire.

Because, it is within embracing these almost enough moments that they become my ever upward, where I can open myself and my life up enough for them to become my *more than enough moments.*

But, it has only been through my sufferings and my fight for recovery that I have been able to really see, let alone embrace, these moments as being more than enough.

This is ever upward.
My recovery.
My story.
My purpose.
My path.
My light.
And even, my soul scars.
Allowing every single almost enough moment to
really be more than enough...this is my ever upward.

Epilogue

March 10th, 2014 my dad fell off a 6 foot ladder while working a job as the heating and cooling contractor. His injuries were extensive, including several skulls fractures (including both walls of the sinus cavity), two brain bleeds, an air pocket on his brain, several facial fractures and a hypoxic seizure. He was admitted to the ICU and I was home for over a week when he first fell. After returning home to my practice, my dogs and real life I realized I had a lot of catch up to play; especially catch up with my recovery.

Life happens; we fall behind in our self care, behind in our recovery, and all of a sudden we are fighting our own gravity of relapse.

The song *Gravity* by Sara Bareilles is powerful in its own right. As a mental health therapist who works with clients struggling with addiction, the power of the lyrics were solidified for me when Mia Michaels choreographed a dance to it on *So You Think You Can Dance* years ago. After my dad's accident, the lyrics hit home as I could feel the pull of old ways on me; the gravity of my own relapse.

Being home helping family meant I didn't make myself, my recovery, a priority. I am the first to admit that recovery is multiple choices I make every single day to be the best version of myself; it is exercise, it is writing, it is meditation, it is reading, it is a nighttime routine, it is expressing myself...it is a huge pain in the ass. But they are daily choices I must make to live my wholehearted recovered life.

I am carefully minding the balance between being gentle with myself in that I did the very best I could given the situation I was in and being frustrated that I didn't fight harder for myself and my recovery. I wasn't in my own home. I was helping during a very stressful time for all of us. I wasn't eating the way I normally do. I was around someone who doesn't believe or honor, and sometimes even actively denies, my story and recovery; one of my biggest incapables. I was way behind on sleep. I did the best I could, but I know now that I need to choose better next time.

Fighting the gravity of relapse, meant that I still made sure to listen to my play list every morning as I got ready. It was the one daily choice of my recovery I made sure to practice even during that stressful time. Fighting the gravity of relapse, meant that I slowly got back on track with my daily choices, adding new ones each day until I was back to what it takes to maintain my ever upward light. Fighting the gravity of relapse, meant asking for help from my loved ones and getting in to see my own therapist the week I got home. Fighting the gravity of relapse, also means doing better next time but giving myself a break on this time. Fighting the gravity of relapse, means giving myself permission that I am always learning, growing and figuring it all out along the way. Fighting the gravity of relapse, means writing this to own my struggle because it is in this ownership that I will find my recovery again and simply take the best next step forward.

Because, it is only within the honoring of this battle that I will make it part of my journey in my ever upward.

Owning my struggle and fight against the gravity of relapse also meant diving head first back into the blog, where I owned my fear and submitted posts to two huge blogs. National Infertility Awareness Week 2014 came and went, I participated some but the timing was not the best just coming out of dad's accident. The theme that year was *Resolve to Know More*. Considering that everything about infertility seems to be anything but clear, both to the general public for the most part and sometimes to those of us in the midst of it I felt compelled to participate.

The gut wrenching and crystal clear part of infertility is that it affects one in eight couples.

And, I am One in Eight.

But, I am one of the one in eight that refuses to stay in my dark, shamed silence.

There are countless ways a family finds themselves seeking further testing or trying assisted fertility treatments; recurrent miscarriage, Polycystic Ovarian Syndrome, Endometriosis, chromosome disorders, physical limitations, medical sterility, unexplained infertility, etc. The paths that lead any of us to the world of infertility treatments are so different and yet can feel so much the same once in the humbling hell of the world of infertility treatments.

The so different and yet the very same theme also carries us straight through the synthetic hormonal hell of infertility treatments. No matter what your protocol looks like, how long it lasts or how many times you try different versions; Clomid, Intrauterine Insemination (IUI), In Vitro Fertilization (IVF), traditional or gestational surrogacy, embryo adoption, adoption, etc. The impossible decisions of infertility are decisions only to be made by each family individually. How much can you physically take? How much can you afford financially? How much can you give up and take emotionally? Ultimately, how far do you have to go in order to be okay with letting go of a lifelong dream?

Each of us will survive through infertility in our very different, and yet I think, very same ways. Some of us will tell absolutely no one besides our partner; the shame and fear and cautious hopefulness feeling like it's just too much to put out there. Some of us will tell everyone, seeking support and opinions, attempting to break the silence and also knowing that this journey is just too difficult to not have as much support as possible. All of us just stumbling forward, trying to figure out how to survive what feels like an impossible journey. Shielding ourselves from judgment and misunderstanding of the impossible decisions we must make. Protecting our hearts from invalidating and minimizing questions every day, from strangers and our loved ones. All while just fighting for what so many take for granted...a family.

Some of us will try for many years. Some of us will only be able to try for a couple of years. Some of us will never get to try multiple rounds of expensive treatments. Some of us will get round after round paid for by insurance. Some of us will stop at IUI. Some of us will stop at IVF. Some of us will just stop.

How our infertility journey eventually ends also seems to be so very different and yet very much the same. There are many different ways for our families to look after infertility. I think the most accepted and expected happy ending is when the treatments work and you end up with a healthy baby, and preferably a sibling, or two or three, one day.

And yet, here I am, recovering and resolving to know my own happy ending, and yet it looks nothing like what is accepted or expected, as I am a child*free* mother.

We must resolve to know that there isn't a perfect answer or ending to infertility. Some of us will get one child, some of us many. Some of these children will be our biological children, some will be adopted and some of us will never get to have children. We will all have scars, especially on our souls, from infertility, no matter the ending. And, we will all have losses and lifelong costs.

We must resolve to know that we must break the silence of infertility. We must own our stories. We must own our impossible decisions. We must give voice to all versions of the happy ending. Because sometimes treatments just aren't going to work. Because sometimes the ending doesn't include children. Because our infertility journeys are so very different, and yet so much the same.

We must resolve to know that once we open ourselves up to all that life has to offer us, children or not, we will find our peace. We will find our recovery. We will find ourselves again in our ever upward happy ending.

• • •

I am not a mother.

I wanted to be a mother.

I fought very hard to be a mother.

I paid a lot of money and put my body (and my surrogate's body) through synthetic hormonal hell to be a mother.

But, I am not a mother, at least in the common definition of mother.

My story could be considered epically sad and tremendously messy. But, I like to think of it as beautifully flawed and filled with ever upward light and love, and every piece of my life puzzle in this messy, beautiful life is proof that I am a warrior. Because, it is messy and beautiful to live our lives authentically brave, and so, every day I choose to live as a Messy, Beautiful Warrior (just as Glennon Melton of Momastery and *Carry On, Warrior* does).

Being a warrior means living all the parts of my story fully, wholeheartedly and brazenly authentically courageous. It means never shying away from the most asked question of every woman my age, "How many children do you have?", and answering it in my own honest way.

"We tried, we tried really hard, but we can't have kids."

It means never allowing shame to steal my story when I am asked the inevitable second most asked question, "Well, why don't you just adopt?"

"We know adoption is not our path. We've been through a lot, financially and emotionally, with In Vitro Fertilization (IVF), surrogacy and losing three babies already. We have decided to accept a childfree life."

I will not apologize if my answer makes you uncomfortable. I will not allow your need to fix or take away my pain to silence my story. I will not let shame, self- or societal-induced, steal my light.

So I will educate. I will write and speak my story, owning my shame, every day of my life. I will live it because it is the only way to honor myself. I will live it because it is the only way the landscape of infertility will change. I will live it because we all have our own epically messy, beautiful journeys. Because hard is hard and maybe, just maybe, openly owning my story will make you just uncomfortable enough to open your eyes and heart to someone else's story and therefore lead you to some compassion and understanding.

In short, Ever Upward is the epitome of messy, beautiful. It is about what happens when we don't get what we so desperately wanted and hoped for. What happens when we don't get what we thought we deserved?

Ever Upward is about letting go of what isn't and embracing a new purpose.

Ever Upward is living and writing about every epic stumble followed every purposeful rise.

My messy is the random anger and bitterness that can over take me at times. My messy is the underlying sadness that comes and goes because I didn't get what I wanted or hoped for. My messy is that in every traditional sense of a woman my age, I won't ever really fit in because I am not a mother. My messy is owning my struggle of recovery. My messy is my courage to own my shame in my childless status.

But, I choose beautiful in my ever upward mess.

My beautiful is surviving failed IVF and surrogacy. My beautiful is accepting and redefining my childfree life. My beautiful is finding my chosen family within the love of our surrogate family especially with their unexpected pregnancy after our failed IVF tries. My beautiful is finding my role in the lives of all our chosen children. My beautiful is having the patience to find my faith again. My beautiful is owning my story, for the world to see, in order to break the silence of infertility but more importantly in claiming my ongoing recovery. My beautiful is knowing that I am a mother in more ways than most are open to considering. My beautiful is in trusting my gut wrenching ironic path to my ever upward light in being a childfree mother.

As, my beautiful is living my light, authentically brave, mess and all, no matter what. Because life in recovery is always a messy, beautiful ever upward journey.

Singing my heart out, holding back tears, as this seems to be what I did for a while in church as I wrestled so much with myself, with trusting and my faith journey, I had one of my first true writer moments. Smack in the middle of the song, I grabbed my bulletin and pen and wrote the title for a blog post and a line from the song down.

The song: Let Our Faith Be Not Alone by Robbie Seay.

The lyrics: "May our hearts be not of stone, give us souls that never close."

As a therapist, I hear terrible things every day from my clients. And, it is not unusual for the thought to cross my mind that someone has every right to stay sick, to stay angry, to *have hearts of stone and closed souls* after what they have been through.

After infertility and the lifelong losses of three babies, I have also felt as if I have three very good enough reasons to allow my heart to become stone and my soul to close.

But what I have learned, and what is ever upward, is this is not meant to be the end of my story. Nor do I want it to be the end of my story; just as I help my clients every single day to make sure that their losses, traumas and tragedies are not their endings either. Because, I also get to hear amazing stories of hope and recovery every single day.

But this recovery requires the choice to choose hope and to do the work.

I will always have the soul scars of infertility and losing my babies. And if I am not careful these scars could very easily harden my heart and close my soul to the amazingness that is this life. As they are forever scars much like the four inch back surgery scar I have. Except, my soul scars are invisible to the outside world, and many times are completely misunderstood, invalidated, minimized and sometimes even ignored.

Either scar, back or soul, if ignored by me only worsens; the scar tissue builds up, increasing the pain and decreasing my quality of life. For my back it is only through my physical therapy, exercise and self care that this old injury and scar tissue can be as healed as possible. Nothing I do will ever make that scar go away, but I sure as hell can make sure I do what is in my power to make it as better as possible. And, almost 20 years later, I wouldn't want that scar to go away anyways, as it is a constant reminder of how much strength I truly hold.

As for my soul scars, I must do much of the same work. If I do not do the work of recovery from the trauma of infertility, the lifelong losses and costs of IVF and the ongoing work of accepting a childfree life, I will only allow the scar tissue to grow. And if I am not careful my heart and soul will scar over leaving room for only bitterness, anger and sadness.

Our trauma, tragedies and losses (infertility related or not) make us who we are. I have learned that I am a better *everything* because I wanted and loved those babies so much. I am also a better everything because I lost them. Sure, the losses left my heart and soul shattered at first, but now with daily work in recovery I have a scarred but healing heart and soul.

Scarred, but better and complete, and most definitely open.

• • •

This openness is not possible without the daily practice of recovery, authentic living and courage. My choices in recovery, in daily practice, and my faith are what is required for me to not allow the scar tissue to close everything. And I did not survive infertility and lose my three dreams to only be left scarred, closed and hardened like stone.

I am still wholeheartedly figuring this whole thing out, awkwardly stumbling through this life in recovery. And, sometimes I am not a very pretty picture while doing it. What I think I am finally coming to terms with and learning is that I can trust that the end of my story isn't supposed to be a heart of stone or a scarred, closed soul. That I can trust my faith, doubts and all, because within this journey I will always have Him[5]. And it is with His acceptance, love and help that I will continue to fight for, find and redefine my *ever upward.*

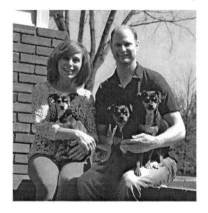

---

5   *For me, my faith is in God and Jesus as my savior. This is something I am newly figuring out, with a lot of doubt and struggle and questions. But it is something that is helping me, especially in my recovery. My only hope is that we can all find something to have faith in.*

Resources

Books

Comfortable with Uncertainty: 108 Teachings on Cultivating Fearlessness and Compassion by Pema Chödrön, Shambhala, 2003.

Daring Greatly by Brené Brown, Gotham, 2012.

Eat Right For Your Type by Peter D'Adamo with Catherine Whitney, Putnam Adult, 1997.

The Gifts of Imperfection by Brené Brown, Hazelden, 2010.

Websites

Brené Brown: http://brenebrown.com/

The Daring Way™: http://thedaringway.com/

Elizabeth Gilbert: http://www.elizabethgilbert.com/

Emerging Women: http://www.emergingwomen.com/

Erin Weed: http://www.erinweed.com/

Eve Ensler: http://www.eveensler.org/

Journeying Beyond Breast Cancer: http://journeyingbeyondbreastcancer.com/

Kelly McGonigal: http://kellymcgonigal.com/
Kristen Neff: http://www.self-compassion.org/
Kristen Wheeler: http://www.kristenwheeler.com
Pharrell Williams, Happy: http://24hoursofhappy.com/
Relationships First: http://relationshipsfirst.org/

Speech

The Man in the Arena, excerpt from Theodore Roosevelt's "Citizenship in a Republic" speech, 1910.

Songs

Just Be Held by Casting Crowns, © 2014 Provident Label Group LLC, a unit of Sony Music Entertainment.
Let Our Faith Be Not Alone by Robbie Seay Band, (C) 2010 Sparrow Records.

The Daring Way™

The Daring Way™ is a highly experiential methodology based on the research of Dr. Brené Brown. The method was developed to help men, women and adolescent learn how to show up, be seen, and live braver lives. The primary focus is on developing shame resilience skills and developing daily practices that transform the way we live, love, parent, and lead. It can be facilitated in clinical, educational or professional setting and is suitable to work with individuals, couples, families and groups.

Brené Brown, PhD, LMSW is a research professor at the University of Houston Graduate College of Social Work. She has spent the past twelve years studying vulnerability, courage, worthiness and shame. Her groundbreaking research has been featured on PBS, NPR, CNN, The Katie Show and Oprah Winfrey's Super Soul Sunday.

Brené is the author of the #1 New York Times bestseller *Daring Greatly: How the Courage to Be Vulnerable Transforms the Way We Live, Love, Parent, and Lead* (2012), The New York Times bestseller *The Gifts of Imperfection* (2010) and *I Thought It Was Just Me* (2007).

Brené's 2010 TEDx Houston talk "The Power of Vulnerability" is one of the top ten most viewed TED talks in the world, with over 11 million viewers. Additionally, Brené gave the closing talk at the 2012 TED conference, where she talked about shame, courage and innovation.

About the Author

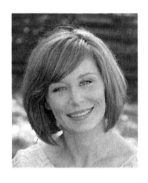

Justine Brooks Froelker a Licensed Professional Counselor and a Certified Daring Way™ Facilitator (based on the research of Brené Brown) with a private practice in St. Louis, Missouri. For the last 14 years she has worked with clients using a combination of Cognitive Behavioral Therapy and Solution Focused Therapy in a straight-forward and non-shaming approach to create a safe space for clients to address concerns. She has extensive experience working with all ages on such concerns as anxiety, depression, relationships, infertility, addictions, perfectionism, eating and weight issues and common discontent.

In addition to Justine's private practice, she is an adjunct faculty member at Saint Louis Community College, where she teaches General Psychology. Additionally, Justine writes as an expert therapist for the monthly publication St. Louis Health & Wellness Magazine. She also can be seen regularly on the St. Louis KMOV live midday show, *Great Day St. Louis.*

In February 2011, Justine and her husband began their journey in the world of IVF. Gestational surrogacy was the safest way for them to have their children since Justine had suffered two back surgeries in high school (including a year of her life spent in a body cast). Two rounds of IVF, two transfers and three babies never to be born later, *Ever Upward* was conceived. After much mourning, confusion, anger and sadness, Justine got back up and started doing the work. The work to redefine; her life, herself, everything. A big part of her journey has been telling her story, and ultimately educating people on how difficult, expensive and painful IVF can be and that sometimes you just don't get the joy of motherhood from it. And telling her story to model, because we need to talk about it! And that yes, sometimes it is okay to say no more. And even more, it is okay to say adoption isn't for you. And that after the work, you can take the step forward into a fulfilled childfree life and stop being stuck in the childless life, even in this, our child obsessed world. *Ever Upward* is not the typical infertility book and blog filled with follicle counts, Clomid crazy train side effects and recounts of painful procedures. It is filled with struggle, hope and recovery, it is a blog about life.

Ever Upward is Justine's story, and yet every woman's story; mother or not, because behind the wall of silence, shame, the smile, and the 'I can do everything' attitude lies millions of women suffering in silence with the pain of infertility. And yet our connection to our stories, is the only way back to the truth of who we are, to own ourselves again.

* This book has been part of my healing process. However, I also hope to help others, even if it is just by knowing you are not alone in the journey of life. This book is not meant to be a how-to or even a sure fire answer to others on what steps they need to take to change their own lives. Rather, it is simply an explanation of how I continue the work. Take what applies to you, or what you think you'd like to try, and leave

the rest. We all have to simply find the strategies that work for us, because only then will we choose the change and do the work to continue it. Ever Upward is about finding your path, accepting your story and fighting for recovery...it is about life. *